The Modigliani Scandal

KEN FOLLETT

First published in Great Britain 1976

Copyright © Zachary Stone, 1976
Introduction copyright © Ken Follett, 1985

This edition first published by Harrap Ltd, 1985
when published in paperback by Fana Scanlan, 1997

The right of Ken Follett to be identified as the author
has been asserted in accordance with the Copyright,
Designs and Patents Act, 1988.

All rights reserved. No part of this publication may be reproduced,
stored in a retrieval system or transmitted, in any form or by any means,
electronic, mechanical, photocopying, recording or otherwise, without the
prior written permission of the copyright owner.

This book is sold subject to the condition that it shall not, by way
of trade or otherwise, be lent, re-sold, hired out or otherwise
circulated without the publisher's prior consent in any form of
binding or cover other than that in which it is published and without a similar
condition including this condition being imposed on the
subsequent purchaser.

Published by Cambridge University Press

© Copyright 2001
31, Great Smith Street,
SW1H 9BU, London UK

ISBN: Cet ouvrage est imprimé en Mongaric 285
ISBN: 2100 1988

ISBN: 1-85578-047-8

Pour les notes en marge du texte
© Larousse, 2014
21, rue du Montparnasse
75283 Paris Cedex 06

HARRAP's® est une marque de Larousse SAS
www.harrap.com

ISBN 978 2 81 870284 0

About the author

Ken Follett was only twenty-seven when he wrote the award-winning novel[1] *Eye of the Needle*, which became an international bestseller. He has since written[2] several equally successful[3] novels including, most recently, *World Without End*, the bestselling sequel[4] to *The Pillars of the Earth*. He is also the author of the non-fiction[5] bestseller *On Wings of Eagles*. Ken Follett lives with his family in London and Hertfordshire.

Visit the Ken Follett website at http://www.ken-follett.com

1. *Le roman qui a été récompensé par de nombreux prix*
2. *Depuis, il a écrit*
3. *ayant connu le même succès*
4. *le best seller qui est la suite*
5. *documentaire*

DIRECTION DE LA PUBLICATION : Carine Girac-Marinier

DIRECTION ÉDITORIALE : Claude Nimmo

NOTES EN MARGE : Patricia Seixas

RÉVISION DES NOTES : Valérie Katzaros

RELECTURE : Joëlle Narjollet

INFORMATIQUE ÉDITORIALE : Marie-Noëlle Tilliette

CONCEPTION GRAPHIQUE : Uli Meindl

MISE EN PAGES : Cynthia Savage

FABRICATION : Rebecca Dubois

Mot de l'Éditeur

Vous aimeriez lire en langue originale, mais le vocabulaire, les expressions figurées ou la syntaxe vous arrêtent parfois ?

Cette collection est faite pour vous !

Vous trouverez en effet, en note dans la marge, une traduction de certains mots et expressions qui vous permettra d'avancer facilement dans votre lecture.

Nous n'avons pas cherché à vous donner une traduction littéraire de l'ouvrage et nous nous sommes parfois écartés du sens littéral pour vous fournir celui qui convient le mieux à l'histoire. Aussi les mots sont-ils traduits dans le contexte du texte original.

Les expressions figées anglaises sont, bien entendu, rendues par une expression équivalente en français.

Les allusions à des réalités culturelles du monde anglo-saxon sont expliquées également dans la marge, pour vous aider à mieux comprendre la trame de l'histoire.

Vous aurez ainsi, en regard du texte original, tout le savoir-faire d'un dictionnaire rien que pour vous et adapté à ce livre !

Notre objectif est de vous mener jusqu'au mot FIN en vous donnant les clés nécessaires à la compréhension du récit.

Laissez-vous gagner par l'angoisse, l'humour et le suspense qui règnent chez les maîtres de la littérature anglo-saxonne.

Lire en VO ? You can indeed!

Contents

Contents

Introduction

In a modern thriller[1] the hero generally saves the world. Traditional adventure stories[2] are more modest: The central character merely saves[3] his own life, and perhaps the life of a faithful friend or a plucky girl[4]. In less sensational novels – the middlebrow, well-told narratives[5] that have been the staple diet of readers[6] for more than a century – there is less at stake[7], but still a character's efforts, struggles[8] and choices determine his destiny in a dramatic fashion[9].

I don't actually[10] believe that life is like that. In reality, circumstances quite beyond our control[11] usually determine whether we live or die, become happy or miserable, strike it rich[12] or lose everything. For example: most rich people inherit their money. Most well-fed[13] people simply had the luck to be born in an affluent country[14]. Most happy people were born into loving families, and most miserable people had crazy parents.

I'm not a fatalist, nor do I believe that everything in life is blind chance[15]. We do not control our lives the way a chess player[16] controls his pieces, but life is not roulette either. As usual, the truth is complicated. Mechanisms beyond our control – and sometimes beyond our understanding[17] – determine a person's fate[18], yet[19] the choices he makes have consequences, if not the consequences he anticipated.

In *The Modigliani Scandal* I tried to write a new kind of novel, one that would reflect[20] the subtle subordination of individual freedom[21] to more

1. roman à suspense d'aujourd'hui

2. récits d'aventures

3. Le héros se contente de sauver

4. une jeune fille audacieuse

5. ces histoires sans prétention et bien racontées

6. le pain quotidien des lecteurs

7. l'enjeu est moindre

8. les épreuves

9. forgent son destin

10. en fait

11. totalement indépendantes de notre volonté

12. faisons fortune

13. bien nourris

14. un pays riche

15. un pur hasard

16. joueur d'échecs

17. incompréhensibles

18. destin

19. néanmoins

20. un roman qui montrerait

21. comment la liberté individuelle dépend, subtilement,

9

1. de rouages qui la dépassent

2. projet prétentieux

3. j'ai échoué

4. ne se limite pas à

5. roman policier léger

6. divers individus, jeunes pour la plupart

7. montent toutes sortes de coups

8. se termine

9. Les critiques ont salué son caractère alerte

10. exubérant

11. enjoué

12. très léger

13. le sérieux de mes intentions

14. je ne considère plus

15. comme un échec

16. C'est un livre léger en effet

17. et cela ne lui enlève rien

18. que je voulais écrire

19. cela prouve plutôt ce que j'avance

powerful machinery[1]. In this immodest project[2] I failed[3]. It may be that such a novel cannot be written: even if Life is not about[4] individual choice, perhaps Literature is.

What I wrote, in the end, was a lighthearted crime story[5] in which an assortment of people, mostly young[6], get up to a variety of capers[7], none of which turns out[8] quite as expected. The critics praised it as sprightly[9], ebullient[10], light, bright, cheery[11], light (again), and fizzy[12]. I was disappointed that they had not noted my serious intentions[13].

Now I no longer look on[14] the book as a failure[15]. It *is* fizzy[16], and none the worse for that[17]. The fact that it is so different from the book I intended to write[18] should not have surprised me. After all, it rather proves my point[19].

KEN FOLLETT, 1985

Coup de pouce pour vous aider à bien comprendre le début de l'histoire...

Nous sommes à Paris où Dee Sleigh, jeune étudiante anglaise en histoire de l'art, vit avec son ami américain et s'apprête à étudier dans une thèse l'influence de la drogue sur l'art. Également dans le milieu de l'art, son ami lui indique le nom d'un vieux monsieur qui aurait bien connu certains des grands maîtres. Or, cette visite va la lancer à la poursuite d'un tableau de Modigliani dont on a perdu la trace...

Part One

Priming the Canvas

'One does not marry art. One ravishes it.'

EDGAR DEGAS,
Impressionist painter

Chapter One

The baker scratched his black moustache with a floury finger[1], turning the hairs grey and unintentionally making himself look ten years older[2]. Around him the shelves[3] and counters were full of long loaves of fresh, crusty bread[4], and the familiar smell filled his nostrils and swelled his chest[5] with a quietly satisfied pride[6]. The bread was a new batch[7], the second that morning: business was good because the weather was fine. He could always rely on[8] a little sunshine to bring the housewives[9] of Paris out into the streets to shop for[10] his good bread.

He looked out of the shop window, narrowing his eyes[11] against the brightness outside. A pretty girl was crossing the street. The baker listened, and heard the sound of his wife's voice, out in the back, arguing shrilly[12] with an employee. The row[13] would go on for several minutes – they always did. Satisfied that he was safe, the baker permitted himself to gaze at the girl lustfully[14].

Her summer dress was thin and sleeveless[15], and the baker thought it looked rather expensive, although he was no expert in such things. The flared skirt swung gracefully[16] at mid-thigh[17], emphasizing her slim bare legs[18], promising – but never quite delivering[19] – delightful glimpses of feminine underwear[20].

She was too slender[21] for his taste, he decided as she came closer. Her breasts were very small – they did not even jiggle[22] with her long, confident

1. le doigt plein de farine
2. se vieillissant de dix ans
3. les rayonnages
4. miches de pain frais et croustillant
5. envahit ses narines et gonfla sa poitrine
6. d'un discret sentiment de fierté
7. fournée
8. compter sur
9. les ménagères
10. acheter
11. en plissant les yeux
12. se disputait d'une voix perçante
13. la querelle
14. contempler la jeune fille d'un œil lubrique
15. sans manches
16. La jupe évasée flottait avec grâce
17. arrivant à mi-cuisse
18. soulignant la finesse de ses jambes nues
19. sans jamais les révéler totalement
20. un délicieux aperçu des dessous féminins
21. mince
22. bougeaient

stride[1]. Twenty years of marriage to Jeanne-Marie had not made the baker tire of plump, pendulous breasts[2].

The girl came into the shop, and the baker realized she was no beauty. Her face was long and thin, her mouth small and ungenerous, with slightly protruding upper teeth[3]. Her hair was brown under a layer of sun-bleached blonde[4].

She selected a loaf from the counter, testing its crust with her long hands, and nodding in satisfaction[5]. No beauty, but definitely desirable, the baker thought.

Her complexion[6] was red-and-white, and her skin looked soft and smooth. But it was her carriage[7] that turned heads. It was confident[8], self-possessed[9]; it told the world that this girl did precisely what she wanted to do, and nothing else. The baker told himself to stop playing with words: she was sexy, and that was that[10].

He flexed his shoulders, to loosen the shirt which was sticking to his perspiring back[11]. '*Chaud, hein?*' he said.

The girl took coins from her purse[12] and paid for her bread. She smiled at his remark, and suddenly she *was* beautiful. '*Le soleil? Je l'aime,*' she said. She closed her purse and opened the shop door. '*Merci!*' she flung over her shoulder[13] as she left.

There had been a trace of accent in her French – an English accent, the baker fancied[14]. But perhaps he had just imagined it to go with her complexion. He stared at her bottom[15] as she crossed the street, mesmerized by the shift[16] of the muscles under the cotton. She was probably returning to the flat of some young, hairy[17] musician, who would still be in bed after a night of debauchery[18].

1. longs pas décidés
2. des seins lourds et charnus
3. les dents du haut légèrement en avant
4. un balayage de mèches blondes
5. en hochant la tête avec satisfaction
6. teint
7. allure
8. pleine d'assurance
9. de maîtrise de soi
10. c'était tout
11. son dos en sueur
12. porte-monnaie
13. lança-t-elle par-dessus son épaule
14. pensa
15. Il regarda ses fesses
16. fasciné par le mouvement
17. chevelu
18. débauche

The shrill voice of Jeanne-Marie approached, shattering the baker's fantasy[1]. He sighed heavily[2], and threw the girl's coins into the till[3].

Dee Sleign smiled to herself[4] as she walked along the pavement away from the shop. The myth was true[5]: Frenchmen were more sensual than Englishmen. The baker's gaze had been candidly lascivious[6], and his eyes had homed in accurately[7] on her pelvis. An English baker would have looked furtively[8] at her breasts from behind his spectacles[9].

She slanted her head back[10] and brushed her hair behind her ears to let the hot sun shine on her face. It was wonderful, this life, this summer in Paris. No work, no exams, no essays, no lectures[11]. Sleeping with Mike[12], getting up late; good coffee and fresh bread for breakfast; days spent[13] with the books she had always wanted to read and the pictures she liked to see; evenings with interesting, eccentric people.

Soon it would be over. Before long she would have to decide what to do with the rest of her life. But for now she was in a personal limbo[14], simply enjoying the things she liked, with no rigid purpose dictating the way she spent every minute.

She turned a corner[15] and entered a small, unpretentious apartment block[16]. As she passed the booth[17] with its tiny window, there was a high-pitched cry[18] from the concierge.

'Mademoiselle!'

The grey-haired woman pronounced each syllable of the word, and managed to give it an accusatory inflection, emphasizing the scandalous fact[19] that Dee was not married to the man who rented[20] the apartment. Dee smiled again; an affair[21] in Paris

1. brisant les fantasmes du boulanger

2. poussa un profond soupir

3. la caisse

4. souriait toute seule

5. La légende était donc vraie

6. Le boulanger l'avait reluquée franchement

7. s'étaient fixés précisément

8. aurait jeté un regard furtif

9. derrière ses lunettes

10. elle pencha la tête en arrière

11. pas de cours

12. Coucher avec Mike

13. des journées passées

14. sur le plan personnel, elle avait mis sa vie entre parenthèses

15. Elle tourna au coin de la rue

16. un petit immeuble quelconque

17. la loge

18. un cri aigu

19. un ton accusateur soulignant qu'il était scandaleux

20. qui louait

21. une liaison

would hardly[1] be complete without a disapproving concierge.

'Télégramme,' the woman said. She laid[2] the envelope on the sill[3] and retired into the cat-smelling gloom of her booth[4], as if to dissociate herself entirely from loose-moralled[5] young girls and their telegrams.

Dee picked it up and ran up the stairs[6]. It was addressed to her, and she knew what it was.

She entered the apartment, and laid the bread and the telegram on the table in the small kitchen. She poured[7] coffee beans into a grinder[8] and pressed the button; the machine growled harshly[9] as it pulverized the brown-black nuts.

Mike's electric shaver whined as if in answer[10]. Sometimes the promise of coffee was the only thing that got him out of bed. Dee made a whole pot[11] and sliced[12] the new bread.

Mike's flat was small, and furnished with elderly stuff of undistinguished taste[13]. He had wanted something more grand[14], and he could certainly afford better[15]. But Dee had insisted they stay out of hotels and classy districts[16]. She had wanted to spend summer with the French, not the international jet set; and she had got her way[17].

The buzz of his shaver died, and Dee poured two cups of coffee.

He came in just as she placed the cups on the round wooden table. He wore his faded, patched Levis[18], and his blue cotton shirt was open at the neck, revealing a tuft of black hair[19] and a medallion on a short silver chain.

'Good morning, darling,' he said. He came round the table and kissed her. She wound her arms around his waist[20] and hugged[21] his body against her own, and kissed him passionately.

'Wow! That was strong for so early in the morning,' he said. He gave a wide California grin[1], and sat down.

Dee looked at the man as he sipped his coffee gratefully[2], and wondered whether she wanted to spend the rest of her life with him. Their affair had been going for a year now[3], and she was getting used to it. She liked his cynicism, his sense of humour, and his buccaneering style[4]. They were both interested in art to the point of obsession, although his interest lay in the money to be made out of it[5], while she[6] was absorbed by the whys and wherefores[7] of the creative process. They stimulated each other, in bed and out: they were a good team.

He got up, poured more coffee, and lit cigarettes for both of them. 'You're quiet,' he said, in his low, gravelly[8] American accent. 'Thinking about those results? It's about time they came through.[9]'

'They came today,' she replied. 'I've been putting off opening the telegram.[10]'

'What? Hey, c'mon, I want to know how you did[11].'

'All right.' She fetched[12] the envelope and sat down again before tearing it open with her thumb. She unfolded the single sheet[13] of thin paper, glanced at it, then looked up at him with a broad smile.

'My God, I got a First[14],' she said.

He leaped to his feet[15] excitedly. 'Yippee!' he yelled. 'I knew it! You're a genius!' He broke into[16] a whining, fast imitation of a country-and-western square dance[17], complete with calls of 'Yee-hah' and the sounds of a steel guitar[18]; and hopped[19] around the kitchen with an imaginary partner.

Dee laughed helplessly. 'You're the most juvenile thirty-nine-year-old I've ever met,' she gasped[20]. Mike bowed in acknowledgement[21] of imaginary applause, and sat down again.

1. Il afficha le grand sourire du Californien
2. tandis qu'il dégustait chaque gorgée de son café
3. Cela faisait un an qu'ils étaient ensemble
4. son allure d'aventurier
5. mais lui s'intéressait surtout à l'argent qu'il pouvait en tirer
6. alors qu'elle
7. le pourquoi du comment
8. rocailleux
9. Il serait temps qu'ils arrivent.
10. Je n'ose pas ouvrir le télégramme.
11. comment tu t'en es sortie
12. elle alla chercher
13. elle déplia l'unique feuillet
14. mention très bien
15. Il se leva d'un bond
16. Il se lança dans
17. une imitation de danse country endiablée
18. [guitare américaine qui se joue à plat]
19. sautilla
20. dit-elle, haletante
21. s'inclina en remerciement

He said: 'So. What does this mean, for your future?'

Dee became serious again. 'It means I get to do[1] my Ph.D[2].'

'What, more degrees[3]? You now have a B.A.[4] in Art History, on top of[5] some kind of Diploma in Fine Art[6]. Isn't it time you stopped being a professional student?'

'Why should I? Learning is my kick[7] – if they're willing[8] to pay me to study for the rest of my life, why shouldn't I do it?'

'They won't pay you much.'

'That's true.' Dee looked thoughtful[9]. 'And I would like to make a fortune[10], somehow[11]. Still, there's plenty of time. I'm only twenty-five.'

Mike reached across the table and held her hand[12]. 'Why don't you come work for me? I'll pay you a fortune – you'd be worth it.'

She shook her head. 'I don't want to ride on your back[13]. I'll make it myself.'

'You're quite happy to ride on my front[14],' he grinned.

She put on a leer.[15] 'You betcha[16],' she said in imitation of his accent. Then she withdrew her hand. 'No, I'm going to write my thesis. If it gets published I could make some cash.'

'What's the topic?'

'Well, I've been toying with a couple of things[17]. The most promising is the relationship between art and drugs.'

'Trendy.[18]'

'And original. I think I could show that drug abuse tends to be[19] good for art and bad for artists.'

'A nice paradox. Where will you start?'

'Here. In Paris. They used to smoke pot[20] in the artistic community around the first couple of decades[21] of the century. Only they called it[22] hashish.'

---

1. je.peux faire
2. [doctorat de 3ᵉ cycle]
3. Quoi, encore des diplômes ?
4. [Bachelor of Arts : licence]
5. en plus de
6. [diplôme des beaux-arts]
7. Faire des études, c'est le pied
8. s'ils veulent bien
9. prit un air pensif
10. gagner beaucoup d'argent
11. d'une manière ou d'une autre
12. étendit le bras et lui prit la main
13. vivre à ta charge
14. de me chevaucher
15. Elle lui jeta un regard concupiscent.
16. Ça, c'est sûr
17. j'hésite entre deux ou trois choses
18. C'est dans l'air du temps.
19. est généralement
20. Ils fumaient de l'herbe
21. les vingt premières années
22. Sauf qu'ils appelaient ça

Mike nodded. 'Will you take[1] just a little help from me, right at the start?'

Dee reached for[2] the cigarettes and took one. 'Sure,' she said.

He held his lighter across the table. 'There's an old guy you ought to talk to[3]. He was a pal of[4] half a dozen of the masters here before World War One[5]. A couple of times he's put me on the track[6] of pictures.

'He was kind of a fringe criminal[7], but he used to get prostitutes to act as models – and other things sometimes – for the young painters. He's old now – he must be pushing ninety[8]. But he remembers.'

*

The tiny bedsitter[9] smelled bad. The odour of the fish shop below pervaded everything[10], seeping up through the bare floorboards[11] and settling in the battered furniture[12], the sheets on the single bed in the corner, the faded curtains[13] at the one small window. Smoke from the old man's pipe failed to hide the fishy smell[14], and underlying it all was the atmosphere of a room that is rarely scrubbed[15].

And a fortune in post-Impressionist paintings hung on the walls.

'All given to me by the artists,' the old man explained airily[16]. Dee had to concentrate to understand his thick Parisian French[17]. 'Always, they were unable to pay their debts. I took the paintings because I knew they would never have the money. I never liked the pictures then[18]. Now I see why they paint this way, and I like it. Besides, they bring back memories.[19]'

The man was completely bald[20], and the skin of his face was loose[21] and pale. He was short[22], and walked with difficulty; but his small black eyes

1. Tu veux bien
2. étendit la main pour prendre
3. un vieil homme à qui tu devrais parler
4. Il était ami avec
5. la Première Guerre mondiale
6. m'a mis sur la piste
7. criminel marginal
8. il doit avoir près de 90 ans
9. chambre meublée
10. L'odeur de la poissonnerie d'en bas imprégnait tout
11. en s'infiltrant par les lames du plancher dépourvues de tapis
12. meubles délabrés
13. rideaux défraîchis
14. ne masquait pas l'odeur de poisson
15. nettoyée à fond
16. avec désinvolture
17. son français au fort accent parisien
18. à cette époque
19. En plus, ils me rappellent des souvenirs.
20. chauve
21. distendue
22. Il était petit

1. pétillaient
parfois
d'enthousiasme

2. Cette jolie
petite Anglaise
le faisait
rajeunir

3. N'êtes-vous
par harcelé

4. Je les prête
toujours
volontiers,
moyennant
paiement

5. Il cligna des
yeux.

6. en levant sa
pipe comme s'il
portait un toast

7. Elle opina
de la tête, avec
complicité.

8. un pot à
tabac

9. un joint

10. les jeunes

11. lécha
le papier à
cigarette et finit
de rouler le joint

12. beaucoup

13. avec ça

14. un dessin au
crayon

15. un croquis
sans doute
esquissé à la
hâte

flashed with occasional enthusiasm[1]. He was rejuvenated by this pretty English girl[2], who spoke such good French and smiled at him as if he was a young man again.

'Don't you get pestered[3] by people wanting to buy them?' Dee asked.

'Not any more. I am always willing to lend them out, at a fee.[4]' His eyes twinkled.[5] 'It pays for my tobacco,' he added, raising his pipe in a gesture like a toast[6].

Dee realized what the other element in the smell was: the tobacco in his pipe was mixed with cannabis. She nodded knowingly.[7]

'Would you like some? I have some papers,' he offered.

'Thank you.'

He passed her a tobacco tin[8], some cigarette papers, and a small block of resin, and she began rolling a joint[9].

'Ah, you young girls,' the man mused. 'Drugs are bad for you, really. I should not corrupt the youth[10]. There, I have been doing it all my life, and now I am too old to change.'

'You've lived a long life on it,' Dee said.

'True, true. I will be eighty-nine this year, I think. For seventy years I have smoked my special tobacco every day, except in prison, of course.'

Dee licked the gummed paper and completed the reefer[11]. She lit it with a tiny gold lighter and inhaled. 'Did the painters use hashish a great deal[12]?' she asked.

'Oh yes. I made a fortune from the stuff[13]. Some spent all their money on it.' He looked at a pencil drawing[14] on the wall, a hurried-looking sketch[15] of the head of a woman; an oval face and a long, thin nose[1]. 'Dedo was the worst[2],' he added with a faraway smile[3].

Dee made out[4] the signature on the drawing. 'Modigliani?'

'Yes.' The man's eyes now saw only the past, and he talked as if to himself[5]. 'He always wore a brown corduroy jacket[6] and a big, floppy felt hat[7]. He used to say that art should be like hashish: it should show people the beauty in things, the beauty they could not normally see. He would drink[8], too, in order to see the ugliness[9] in things. But he loved the hashish.

'It was sad that he had such a conscience about it. I believe he was brought up quite strictly[10]. Also, his health[11] was a little delicate, so he worried about the drugs. He worried, but he still used them.' The old man smiled and nodded, as if agreeing with his memories[12].

'He lived at the Impasse Falguière. He was so poor; he grew haggard[13]. I remember when he went to the Egyptian section in the Louvre – he came back saying it was the only section worth seeing[14]!' He laughed happily. 'A melancholy man, though,' he went on, his voice sobering[15]. 'He always had *Les Chants de Maldoror* in his pocket: he could recite many French verses. The Cubism arrived at the end of his life. It was alien to him.[16] Perhaps it killed him.'

Dee spoke softly, to guide the old man's memory without dislocating his train of thought[17]. 'Did Dedo ever paint while he was high[18]?'

The man laughed lightly. 'Oh yes,' he said. 'While he was high he would paint very fast, shouting all the time that this would be his masterpiece, his *chef-d'œuvre*, that now all Paris would see what painting was all about. He would choose the brightest[19] colours and throw them at the canvas[20]. His friends

1. un nez fin et long

2. le pire de tous

3. un sourire lointain

4. déchiffra

5. comme s'il s'adressait à lui-même

6. une veste en velours côtelé marron

7. chapeau en feutre mou

8. Il buvait

9. la laideur

10. élevé de façon très stricte

11. sa santé

12. comme s'il adhérait à ses souvenirs

13. il allait de plus en plus mal

14. qui valait la peine d'être vue

15. d'une voix plus apaisée

16. Cela lui était étranger.

17. le fil de sa pensée

18. lorsqu'il était défoncé

19. les plus éclatantes

20. les projetait sur la toile

1. que son œuvre ne valait rien
2. d'aller au diable
3. Une fois revenu à son état normal,
4. Il tira sur sa pipe
5. allumettes
6. Le charme était rompu.
7. chaise droite
8. Il raviva sa pipe en tirant des bouffées
9. se renfonça dans son fauteuil
10. Les bouffées successives
11. le replongèrent progressivement dans
12. loyer
13. propriétaire
14. Il y avait à peine assez de place
15. encore moins pour
16. prêtait
17. grommela
18. un pincement de douleur
19. brouette
20. une cour
21. y met le feu
22. il devait trop d'argent
23. j'ai regretté de ne pas lui en avoir prêté
24. de sa période haschich
25. grand feu
26. Dee chuchotait presque
27. Presque tous.

would tell him the work was useless[1], terrible, and he would tell them to piss off[2], they were too ignorant to know that this was the painting of the twentieth century. Then, when he came down,[3] he would agree with them, and throw the canvas in the corner.' He sucked at his pipe[4], noticed it had gone out, and reached for matches[5]. The spell was broken.[6]

Dee leaned forward in her hard upright chair[7], the joint between her fingers forgotten. There was a low intensity in her voice.

She said: 'What happened to those paintings?'

He puffed his pipe into life[8] and leaned back[9], drawing on it rhythmically. The regular suck, puff, suck, puff[10], drew him gradually back into[11] his reverie. 'Poor Dedo,' he said. 'He could not pay the rent[12]. He had nowhere to go. His landlord[13] gave him twenty-four hours to get out. He tried to sell some paintings, but the few people who could see how good they were had no more money than he.

'He had to move in with one of the others – I forget who. There was hardly room[14] for Dedo, let alone[15] his paintings. The ones he liked, he loaned[16] to close friends.

'The rest—' the old man grunted[17], as if the memory had given him a twinge of pain[18]. 'I see him now, loading them into a wheelbarrow[19] and pushing them down the street. He comes to a yard[20], piles them up in the centre, and sets fire to them[21]. "What else is there to do?" he keeps saying. I could have lent him money, I suppose, but he owed too much[22] already. Still, when I saw him watch his paintings burning, I wished I had[23]. There, I was never a saint, in my youth any more than in my old age.'

'All the hashish[24] paintings were on that bonfire[25]?' Dee's voice was almost a whisper.[26]

'Yes,' the old man said. 'Virtually all of them.[27]'

'Virtually? He kept some?'

'No, he kept none[1]. But he had given some to somebody – I had forgotten, but talking to you brings it back[2]. There was a priest[3], in his home town[4], who took an interest in Oriental drugs. I forget why – their medicinal value[5], their spiritual properties? Something like that. Dedo confessed his habits[6] to the priest, and was granted absolution[7]. Then the priest asked to see the work he did under the influence of hashish[8]. Dedo sent him a painting – only one, I remember now.'

The reefer burned Dee's fingers, and she dropped it in an ashtray[9]. The old man lit his pipe again, and Dee stood up.

'Thank you very much for talking to me,' she said.

'Mmm.' Half of the man's mind was still in the past. 'I hope it helps you with your thesis,' he said.

'It certainly has,' she said. On impulse[10] she bent over the man's chair and kissed his bald head. 'You've been kind.'

His eyes twinkled. 'It's a long time since a[11] pretty girl kissed me,' he said.

'Of all the things you've told me, that's the only one I disbelieve[12],' replied Dee. She smiled at him again, and went out through the door.

She controlled her jubilation as she walked along the street. What a break![13] And before she had even started the new term[14]! She was bursting to tell someone about it. Then she remembered – Mike had gone: flown to London[15] for a couple of days. Who could she tell?

On impulse, she bought a postcard[16] at a café. She sat down with a glass of wine to write it. The picture showed[17] the café itself, and a view of the street she was in[18].

1. il n'en a gardé aucun

2. mais maintenant qu'on en parle, ça me revient

3. Il y avait un prêtre

4. sa ville natale

5. vertus médicales

6. son accoutumance

7. qui lui accorda l'absolution

8. sous l'emprise du haschich

9. un cendrier

10. Dans un élan

11. Il y a bien longtemps qu'une

12. que je ne crois pas

13. Quel coup de chance !

14. la rentrée

15. il avait pris l'avion pour Londres

16. une carte postale

17. représentait

18. une vue de la rue dans laquelle elle se trouvait

She sipped her *vin ordinaire* and wondered who to write to[1]. She ought to let the family know[2] her results, too. Her mother would be pleased[3], in her vague kind of way, but she really wanted her daughter[4] to be a member of the dying polite society[5] of ball-goers[6] and dressage-riders[7]. She would not appreciate the triumph of a first-class degree[8]. Who would?

Then she realized who would be most delighted[9] for her.

She wrote:

Dear Uncle Charles,
Believe it or not,[10] I got a First! ! ! Even more incredible[11], I am now on the track[12] of a lost Modigliani! ! !

Love,
D.

She bought a stamp[13] for the card and posted it on her way back to[14] Mike's apartment.

Chapter Two

The glamour had gone out of life[1], Charles Lampeth reflected as he relaxed in his Queen Anne[2] dining chair[3]. This place, the house of his friend, had once seen the kind of parties and balls which now happened only in high-budget historical movies. At least two Prime Ministers had dined[4] in this very room[5], with its long oak[6] table and matching panelled walls[7]. But the room, the house, and their owner[8], Lord Cardwell, belonged to a dying race[9].

Lampeth selected a cigar from the box proffered by the butler[10], and allowed the servant to light it[11]. A sip[12] of remarkably old brandy[13] completed his sense of well-being. The food had been splendid, the wives of the two men had retired in the old-fashioned way[14], and now they would talk.

The butler lit Cardwell's cigar and glided out[15]. The two men puffed contentedly for a while[16]. They had been friends for too long for silence to be an embarrassment between them. Eventually[17] Cardwell spoke.

'How is the art market?' he said.

Lampeth gave a satisfied smile. 'Booming, as it has been for years,' he said.

'I've never understood the economics of it[18],' Cardwell replied. 'Why is it so buoyant[19]?'

'It's complex, as you would expect[20],' Lampeth replied. 'I suppose it started when the Americans became art-conscious[21], just before the Second World War. It's the old supply-and-demand mechanism[22]:

1. La belle époque était révolue
2. [style de mobilier anglais de 1702–1714]
3. chaise de salle à manger
4. deux Premier ministre avaient diné
5. dans cette même pièce
6. en chêne
7. ses boiseries réalisées dans la même essence
8. propriétaire
9. une classe en voie de disparition
10. que lui présentait le majordome
11. laissa le domestique le lui allumer
12. Une gorgée
13. cognac
14. selon la tradition
15. s'éclipsa
16. avec plaisir pendant un moment
17. Finalement,
18. les rouages financiers de ce métier
19. dynamique
20. comme on peut s'en douter
21. ont commencé à s'intéresser à l'art
22. la bonne vieille loi de l'offre et de la demande

1. [Maîtres anciens, Europe, XIIIᵉ–XVIIIᵉ s.]

2. sont montés en flèche

3. se sont tournés vers les peintres modernes

4. c'est là que tu as commencé

5. il était difficile

6. sont arrivés

7. ont gagné une fortune

8. Il desserra son nœud papillon

9. acheter des actions ou miser sur un cheval

10. Si on parie sur un grand favori

11. la cote est faible

12. une valeur de premier ordre

13. donc, quand tu vends, le profit est faible

14. tu es sûr

15. a atteint des sommets

16. mèches

17. À combien estimes-tu ma collection aujourd'hui ?

18. dit Lampeth, en fronçant ses sourcils noirs

19. qui se rejoignirent au-dessus de son nez

20. d'abord

the prices of the Old Masters[1] went through the roof[2].

'There weren't enough Old Masters to go around, so people started turning to the moderns[3].'

Cardwell interrupted: 'And that's where you came in[4].'

Lampeth nodded, and sipped appreciatively at his brandy. 'When I opened my first gallery, just after the war, it was a struggle[5] to sell anything painted after 1900. But we persisted. A few people liked them, prices rose gradually, and then the investors moved in[6]. That was when the Impressionists went through the roof.'

'A lot of people made a pile[7],' Cardwell commented.

'Fewer than you think,' said Lampeth. He loosened his bow tie[8] under his double chin. 'It's rather like buying shares or backing horses[9]. Bet on a near-certainty[10], and you find everyone else has backed it, so the odds are low[11]. If you want a blue-chip share[12], you pay a high price for it, so your gain when you sell is marginal[13].

'So with paintings: buy a Velázquez, and you are bound[14] to make money. But you pay so much for it, that you have to wait several years for a fifty per cent gain. The only people who have made fortunes are the ones who bought the pictures they liked, and found that they had good taste when the value of their collections rocketed[15]. People like yourself.'

Cardwell nodded, and the few strands[16] of white hair on his head waved in the slight breeze caused by the movement. He pulled at the end of his long nose. 'What do you think my collection is worth now?[17]'

'Lord.' Lampeth frowned, drawing his black brows[18] together at the bridge of his nose[19]. 'It would depend on how it was sold, for one thing[20]. For another[1], an accurate[2] valuation would be a week's work for an expert.'

'I'll settle for an inaccurate one[3]. You know the pictures – you bought most of them yourself for me.'

'Yes.' Lampeth pictured in his mind[4] the twenty or thirty paintings in the house, and assigned rough values to them[5]. He closed his eyes and added up the sums.

'It must be a million pounds,' he said eventually.

Cardwell nodded again. 'That's the figure[6] I arrived at,' he said. 'Charlie, I need a million pounds.'

'Good Lord!' Lampeth sat upright in his chair. 'You can't think[7] of selling your collection.'

'I'm afraid it has come to that[8],' Cardwell said sadly. 'I had hoped to leave it to the nation, but the realities of business life come first. The company is overstretched[9], there must be a big capital injection within twelve months[10] or it goes to the wall. You know I've been selling off bits of the estate[11] for years, to keep me in this stuff.' He raised his brandy balloon and drank.

'The young blades[12] have caught up with me at last[13],' he went on. 'New brooms sweeping through the financial world.[14] Our methods are outdated. I shall get out as soon as the company is strong enough to hand over[15]. Let a young blade take it on.'

The note of weary[16] despair in his friend's voice angered Lampeth. 'Young blades,' he said contemptuously. 'Their time of reckoning will come.[17]'

Cardwell laughed lightly. 'Now, now, Charlie. My father was horrified when I announced my intention of going into the City. I remember him telling me: "But you're going to inherit the title[18]!" as if that precluded[19] any notion of my touching real money. And you – what did your father say when you opened an art gallery?'

1. Ensuite
2. précise
3. Je me contenterai d'une évaluation imprécise
4. visualisa de mémoire
5. leur affecta des valeurs approximatives
6. chiffre
7. Tu ne songes pas sérieusement
8. Je crains d'être contraint de le faire
9. à la limite de ses capacités financières
10. dans les douze mois
11. je vends des petits bouts de mon patrimoine
12. les jeunes requins
13. ont fini par me rattraper
14. Du sang neuf inonde le monde financier.
15. pour être cédée
16. las
17. Un jour, ils devront vendre des comptes.
18. hériter de mon titre de noblesse
19. excluait

Lampeth acknowledged the point[1] with a reluctant[2] smile. 'He thought it was a namby-pamby occupation[3] for a soldier's son.'

'So, you see, the world belongs[4] to the young blades. So, sell my pictures, Charlie.'

'The collection will have to be broken up[5], to get the best price.'

'You're the expert. No point in my being sentimental about it.[6]'

'Still[7], some of it ought to be kept together for an exhibition[8]. Let's see: a Renoir, two Degas, some Pissarros, three Modiglianis . . . I'll have to think about it. The Cézanne will have to go to auction[9], of course.'

Cardwell stood up, revealing himself to be very tall, an inch or two over six feet[10]. 'Well, let's not linger over the corpse[11]. Shall we join the ladies?'

The Belgrave Art Gallery had the air of a rather superior provincial museum. The hush was almost tangible[12] as Lampeth entered, his black toecapped shoes treading[13] silently on the plain[14], olive-green carpet. At ten o'clock the gallery had only just opened, and there were no customers. Nevertheless, three assistants in black-and-stripes[15] hovered attentively[16] around the reception area.

Lampeth nodded to them and walked through the ground-floor[17] gallery, his expert eye surveying the pictures on the walls as he passed. Someone had hung a modern abstract[18] incongruously next to a primitive[19], and he made a mental note to get it moved[20]. There were no prices on the works: a deliberate policy[21]. People had the feeling that any mention of cash would be greeted with a disapproving frown[22] from one of the elegantly dressed assistants. In order to maintain their self-esteem[1], patrons[2] would tell themselves that they, too, were part of this world where money was a mere detail[3], as insignificant as the date on the cheque. So they spent more. Charles Lampeth was a businessman first, and an art lover second.

He walked up the broad staircase[4] to the first floor, and caught sight of his reflection in the glass of a frame[5]. His tie-knot[6] was small, his collar crisp[7], his Savile Row suit a perfect fit[8]. It was a pity he was overweight[9], but he still cut an attractive figure[10] for his age. He straightened his shoulders reflectively.[11]

He made another mental note: the glass in that frame ought to be non-reflective. There was a pen drawing[12] underneath it – whoever hung it[13] had made a mistake.

He walked to his office, where he hooked his umbrella on the coat-stand[14]. He walked to the window and looked out on to Regent Street while he lit his first cigar of the day. He watched the traffic, making a list in his mind of the things he would have to attend to[15] between now and the first gin and tonic at five o'clock.

He turned around as his junior partner, Stephen Willow, walked in. 'Morning, Willow,' he said, and sat down at his desk.

Willow said: 'Morning, Lampeth.' They stuck to the habit of surnames[16], despite the six or seven years they had been together. Lampeth had brought Willow in to extend the Belgrave's range[17]: Willow had built up a small gallery of his own[18] by nurturing relationships[19] with half-a-dozen young artists who had turned out to be winners. Lampeth had seen the Belgrave lagging slightly behind[20] the market at the time, and Willow had offered a quick way to catch up[21] with the contemporary scene.

1. Pour préserver leur amour-propre
2. les clients
3. n'était qu'un détail
4. le grand escalier
5. aperçut son reflet dans le verre d'un cadre
6. nœud de cravate
7. son col était impeccable
8. costume de Savile Row tombait parfaitement
9. enrobé
10. sa silhouette était encore attirante
11. redressa les épaules, l'air songeur.
12. un dessin au stylo
13. celui qui l'avait installé
14. accrocha son parapluie au portemanteau
15. dont il devait s'occuper
16. Ils s'appelaient toujours par leur nom de famille
17. développer la collection de la galerie Belgrave
18. avait monté sa propre petite galerie
19. en cultivant des relations
20. était légèrement à la traîne
21. de rattraper le décalage

The partnership worked well: although there was a good ten or fifteen years between the two men, Willow had the same basic qualities[1] of artistic taste and business sense as Lampeth.

The younger man laid a folder[2] on the table and refused a cigar. 'We must talk about Peter Usher,' he said.

'Ah, yes. There's something wrong there[3], and I don't know what it is.'

'We took him over[4] when the Sixty-Nine Gallery went broke[5],' Willow began. 'He had done well[6] there for a year – one canvas went for[7] a thousand. Most of them were selling for upwards of five hundred[8]. Since he came to us, he's only sold a couple.'

'How are we pricing?[9]'

'The same range[10] as the Sixty-Nine.'

'They may have been doing naughty things, mind[11],' said Lampeth.

'I think they were. A suspicious number of highly priced[12] pictures reappeared shortly after[13] they had been sold.'

Lampeth nodded. It was the art world's worst-kept secret[14] that dealers sometimes bought their own pictures in order to stimulate demand for a young artist.

Lampeth said: 'And then again[15], you know, we're not the right gallery for Usher.' He saw his partner's raised eyebrows[16], and added: 'No criticism intended[17], Willow – at the time he appeared to be a scoop. But he is very avant-garde, and it probably did him a little damage[18] to become associated with such a respectable gallery as ours. However, that's all in the past[19]. I still think he's a remarkably good young painter, and we owe him our best efforts[20].'

Willow changed his mind[21] about the cigar, and took one from the box on Lampeth's inlaid desk[22].

'Yes, that was my thinking[1]. I've sounded him out[2] about a show[3]: he says he has enough new work to justify it.'

'Good. The New Room, perhaps?' The gallery was too big for it all to be devoted[4] to the work of a single living artist[5], so one-man exhibitions were held[6] in smaller galleries or in part of the Regent Street premises[7].

'Ideal.'

Lampeth mused[8]: 'I still wonder whether we wouldn't be doing him a favour[9] by letting him go elsewhere.'

'Perhaps, but the outside world wouldn't see it like that.'

'You're quite right.'

'Shall I tell him it's on[10], then?'

'No, not yet. There may be something bigger in the pipeline.[11] Lord Cardwell gave me dinner[12] last night. He wants to sell his collection.'

'Ye Gods – the poor chap.[13] That's a tall order for us.[14]'

'Yes, and we shall have to do it carefully. I'm still thinking about it. Leave that slot open for a while[15]'

Willow looked towards the window out of a corner of his eye[16] – a sign, Lampeth knew, that he was straining his memory[17]. 'Hasn't Cardwell got two or three Modiglianis?' he said eventually.

'That's right.' It was no surprise to Lampeth that Willow knew it: part of a top art dealer's job was to know where hundreds of paintings were, who they belonged to, and how much they were worth.

'Interesting,' Willow continued. 'I had word[18] from Bonn yesterday, after you had left. A collection of Modigliani's sketches is on the market[19].'

'What sort?[20]'

1. c'est ce que je pensais
2. Je lui ai demandé son avis
3. exposition
4. pour la consacrer tout entière
5. artiste vivant
6. les expositions dédiées à un seul artiste avaient lieu
7. les locaux de Regent Street
8. réfléchit
9. si on ne lui rendrait pas service
10. que c'est d'accord
11. On a peut-être quelque chose de plus important en vue.
12. m'a invité à dîner
13. Ciel, le pauvre homme.
14. C'est une grosse mission pour nous.
15. Laissez ce créneau ouvert pour l'instant
16. du coin de l'œil
17. qu'il sondait sa mémoire
18. J'ai eu des nouvelles
19. est à vendre
20. De quel genre ?

'Pencil sketches[1], for sculptures. They aren't on the open market[2] yet, of course. We can have them if we want them.'

'Good. We'll buy them anyway – I think Modigliani is due for a rise in value[3]. He's been underrated for a while[4], you know, because he doesn't fit into a neat category[5].'

Willow stood up. 'I'll get on to my contact[6] and tell him to buy. And if Usher enquires[7], I'll stall him[8].'

'Yes. Be nice to him.'

Willow went out, and Lampeth pulled towards him a wire tray[9] containing the morning's post[10]. He picked up an envelope, its top slit ready for him[11] – then his eye fell on a postcard underneath. He dropped the envelope and picked up the postcard. He looked at the picture on the front, and guessed it to be of a street in Paris. Then he turned it over[12] and read the message. He smiled at first, amused by the breathless prose[13] and the forest of exclamation marks[14].

Then he sat back and thought. His niece had a way of giving the impression she was a feminine, scatty young thing[15]; but she had a very sharp brain[16] and a certain cool determination[17]. She usually meant what she said, even if she sounded like a flapper of the 1920s[18].

Lampeth left the rest of his post in the tray, slipped the postcard into his inside jacket pocket, picked up his umbrella, and went out.

Everything about the agency was discreet – even its entrance. It was cleverly designed so that when a taxi drew up in its forecourt[19], the visitor could not be seen from the street as he got out, paid his fare[20], and entered by the door in the side of the portico[21].

The staff, with their mannered subservience[1], were rather like those at the gallery – although for different reasons. If forced to say exactly what the agency's business was, they would murmur that it made enquiries on behalf of its clients[2]. Just as the assistants at the Belgrave never mentioned money, so those at the agency never mentioned detectives.

Indeed, Lampeth had never to his knowledge[3] seen a detective there. The detectives at Lipsey's did not reveal who their clients were for the simple reason that they frequently did not know. Discretion mattered even more than a successful conclusion to an operation[4].

Lampeth was recognized, although he had only been there two or three times. His umbrella was taken, and he was shown into the office[5] of Mr Lipsey: a short, dapper[6] man, with straight black hair, and the slightly mournful, tactfully persistent approach[7] of a coroner at an inquest[8].

He shook hands with Lampeth and motioned him to[9] a chair. His office looked more like a solicitor's[10] than a detective's, with dark wood, drawers instead of filing cabinets[11], and a safe[12] in a wall. His desk was full, but neat, with pencils arranged in a row[13], papers piled tidily[14], and a pocket electronic calculator.

The calculator reminded Lampeth that most of the agency's business[15] involved investigating possible fraud[16]: hence its location[17] in the City. But they also traced individuals and – for Lampeth – pictures. Their fees[18] were high, which gave Lampeth comfort.

'A glass of sherry[19]?' Lipsey offered.

'Thank you.' Lampeth took the postcard from his pocket while the other man poured from a decanter[20]. He took the proffered[21] glass and gave the post-

1.	Les employés, obligeants, aux manières irréprochables
2.	des enquêtes pour le compte de ses clients
3.	à sa connaissance
4.	qu'une opération réussie
5.	on le fit entrer dans le bureau
6.	soigné
7.	cet abord poli et insistant, un peu triste,
8.	du médecin légiste à une audience judiciaire
9.	lui indiqua
10.	au bureau d'un avocat
11.	avec des tiroirs au lieu de classeurs
12.	un coffre-fort
13.	une rangée de crayons bien alignés
14.	soigneusement empilés
15.	les activités de l'agence
16.	d'enquêter sur d'éventuelles fraudes
17.	c'est pourquoi elle était située
18.	honoraires
19.	xérès
20.	carafe
21.	qu'on lui tendait

1. posa son xérès, intact, sur le bureau
2. J'imagine
3. Je vais vous la procurer.
4. à l'heure qu'il est
5. en quête du
6. À moins qu'il ne soit
7. Ce qui fait que nous n'avons que l'adresse de ses amis
8. qu'elle ait flairé la piste, pour ainsi dire
9. formidable découverte
10. C'est fort probable
11. Bien vu.
12. les probabilités
13. qu'on découvre que c'est une fausse piste
14. haussa les épaules
15. ne vous méprenez pas sur la prose de Delia
16. perspicace
17. pour l'empêcher d'aller chez mes concurrents
18. disponible
19. Nous pouvons nous y mettre
20. comment formuler
21. que je suis à l'origine de cette enquête
22. vous vous en doutez bien?

card in exchange. Lipsey sat down, set his sherry untouched on the desk[1] and studied the card.

A minute later he said: 'I take it[2] you want us to find the picture.'

'Yes.'

'Hmm. Do you have your niece's address in Paris?'

'No, but my sister – her mother – will know. I'll get it for you.[3] However, if I know Delia, she will probably have left Paris by now[4] – in search of[5] the Modigliani. Unless it's[6] in Paris.'

'So – we are left with her friends[7] there. And this picture. Is it possible that she got the scent, so to speak[8], of this great find[9] somewhere near the café?'

'That's very likely[10],' said Lampeth. 'Good guessing.[11] She's an impulsive girl.'

'I imagined so from the – ah – style of the correspondence. Now, what are the chances[12] that this will turn out to be a wild goose chase[13]?'

Lampeth shrugged[14]. 'There is always that possibility with searches for lost pictures. But don't be misled by Delia's style[15] – she's just won a First in Art History, and she is a shrewd[16] twenty-five-year-old. If she would work for me I'd employ her, if only to keep her out of the hands of my competitors[17].'

'And the chances?'

'Fifty-fifty. No, better – seventy-thirty. In her favour.'

'Good. Well, I have the right man for the job available[18] at the moment. We can get on to it[19] immediately.'

Lampeth stood up, hesitated, and frowned, as if he did not quite know how to put[20] what he was about to say. Lipsey waited patiently.

'Ah – it's important that the girl should not know that I have initiated the enquiry[21], you realize?[22]'

'Of course,' Lipsey said smoothly. 'It goes without saying.[1]'

The gallery was full of people chatting, clinking glasses[2], and dropping cigar ash[3] on the carpet. The reception was to publicize[4] a small collection of various German Expressionists[5] which Lampeth had acquired in Denmark: he disliked the paintings, but they were a good buy[6]. The people were clients, artists, critics, and art historians. Some had come simply to be seen at the Belgrave, to tell the world that this was the kind of circle they moved in[7]; but they would buy, eventually, to prove that they did not come merely to be seen[8] there. Most of the critics would write about the show, for they could not afford to ignore anything the Belgrave did. The artists came for the canapés and the wine – free food and drink, and some of them needed it. Perhaps the only people who were genuinely interested[9] in the paintings were the art historians and a few serious collectors[10].

Lampeth sighed, and looked furtively at his watch. It would be another hour[11] before he could respectably leave. His wife had long ago given up attending[12] gallery receptions. She said they were a bore[13], and she was right. Lampeth would like to be at home now, with a glass of port[14] in one hand and a book in the other; sitting on his favourite chair – the old leather[15] one, with the hard horsehair upholstery[16] and the burn mark on the arm[17] where he always put his pipe – with his wife opposite[18] him and Siddons coming in to make up the fire[19] for the last time.

1. Cela va sans dire.

2. qui bavardaient et entrechoquaient leurs verres
3. laissaient tomber les cendres de leur cigare
4. Le but de la réception était de faire connaître
5. expressionnistes allemands
6. une bonne affaire
7. le genre de cercle dans lequel ils évoluaient
8. uniquement pour être vus
9. réellement intéressés
10. collectionneurs
11. Il devait patienter encore une heure
12. avait cessé d'assister depuis longtemps
13. ennuyeuses
14. porto
15. en cuir
16. rembourré avec du crin de cheval
17. la trace de brûlure sur l'accoudoir
18. sa femme en face de lui
19. pour remettre du bois dans le feu

'Wishing you were home, Charlie?' The voice came from beside him and broke his daydream[1]. 'Rather[2] be sitting in front of the telly[3] watching Barlow[4]?'

Lampeth forced a smile. He rarely watched television, and he resented being called[5] Charlie by any but his oldest friends[6]. The man he smiled at was not even a friend: he was the art critic of a weekly journal[7], perceptive enough about art[8], especially sculpture, but a terrible bore[9]. 'Hello, Jack, glad you could come,' Lampeth said. 'Actually, I am a bit tired for this sort of bash[10].'

'Know how you feel,' the critic said. 'Hard day? Tough time knocking some poor painter's price down[11] a couple of hundred[12]?'

Lampeth forced another smile, but deigned to reply to the jocular insult[13]. The journal was a left-wing one[14], he remembered, and it felt the need to be disapproving of anyone who actually made money out of culture.

He saw Willow easing through the crowd[15] towards him, and felt gratitude towards his junior partner. The journalist seemed to sense this[16], and excused himself.

'Thank you for rescuing me,' Lampeth said to Willow in a low voice.

'No trouble, Lampeth. What I actually came to say was, Peter Usher is here. Do you want to handle him[17] yourself?'

'Yes. Listen, I've decided to do a Modigliani show. We've got Lord Cardwell's three, the sketches, and another possibility came up this morning. That's enough for a nucleus.[18] Will you find out[19] who's got what?'

'Of course. That means Usher's one-man has had it[20].'

'I'm afraid so. There isn't another slot[1] for that sort of thing for months. I'll tell him. He won't like it, but it won't harm him all that much. His talent will tell in the long run[2], whatever we do.'

Willow nodded and moved away[3], and Lampeth went in search[4] of Usher. He found him at the far end[5] of the gallery, sitting in front of some of the new paintings. He was with a woman, and they had filled a tray[6] with food from the buffet.

'May I join you?' Lampeth said.

'Of course. The sandwiches are delicious,' Usher said. 'I haven't had caviar for days.'

Lampeth smiled at the sarcasm, and helped himself[7] to a tiny square of white bread. The woman said: 'Peter tries to play the part[8] of the angry young man, but he's too old.'

'You haven't met my mouthy wife, have you[9]?' Usher said.

Lampeth nodded. 'Delighted,' he said. 'We're used to Peter[10], Mrs Usher. We tolerate his sense of humour because we like his work so much.'

Usher accepted the rebuke gracefully[11], and Lampeth knew he had put it in exactly the right way[12]: disguised in good manners and larded with flattery[13].

Usher washed another sandwich down with the wine[14], and said: 'When are you going to put on[15] my one-man show, then?'

'Now, that is really what I wanted to talk to you about,' Lampeth began. 'I'm afraid we're going to have to postpone it.[16] You see—'

Usher interrupted him, his face reddening[17] behind the long hair and Jesus beard[18]. 'Don't make phoney excuses[19] – you've found something better to fill the slot. Who is it?'

1. Il n'y a pas d'autre créneau

2. Il a du talent, il finira par percer

3. acquiesça et s'éloigna

4. partit à la recherche

5. tout au bout

6. rempli un plateau

7. se servit

8. de jouer le rôle

9. Je vous présente ma femme, qui est très bavarde

10. Nous connaissons bien Peter

11. accepta le reproche de bonne grâce

12. il l'avait présenté exactement comme il fallait

13. et flatteur par ailleurs

14. avala un autre sandwich, qu'il arrosa de vin

15. organiser

16. Je crains que nous ne soyons contraints de la reporter.

17. le visage empourpré

18. sa barbe fournie

19. des excuses bidon

Lampeth sighed. He had wanted to avoid[1] this. 'We're doing a Modigliani exhibition. But that's not the only—'

'How long?' Usher demanded, his voice louder[2]. His wife put a restraining hand on his arm[3]. 'How long do you propose to postpone my show?'

Lampeth felt eyes boring into his back[4], and guessed that some of the crowd were now watching the scene. He smiled, and inclined his head conspiratorially[5], to try and make Usher talk quietly. 'Can't say,' he murmured. 'We have a very full schedule. Hopefully[6] early next year—'

'Next year!' Usher shouted. 'Jesus Christ, Modigliani can do without[7] a show but I have to live! My family have to eat!'

'Please, Peter—'

'No! I won't shut up!' The whole gallery was quiet now, and Lampeth realized despairingly[8] that everyone was watching the quarrel[9]. Usher yelled[10]: 'I've no doubt you'll make more money out of Modigliani[11], because he's dead. You won't do any good to the human race[12], but you'll make a bomb. There are too many fat profiteers[13] like you running the business[14], Lampeth.

'Do you realize the prices I used to get before I joined this bloody stuffed-shirt gallery[15]? I took out a bloody mortgage on the strength of it[16] All the Belgrave has done is to lower my prices and hide my pictures away so nobody buys them. I've had it with you[17], Lampeth! I'll take my work elsewhere, so stuff your fucking gallery right up your arse[18]!'

Lampeth cringed[19] at the violent language[20]. He was blushing bright red, he knew, but there was nothing he could do about it.

Usher turned theatrically[21] and stormed out[22]. The crowd made a gap for him[23], and he walked through it, his head held high[1]. His wife followed behind, running to keep up[2] with his long-legged stride[3], avoiding the eyes[4] of the guests. Everyone looked at Lampeth for guidance.

'I apologize for[5]... this,' he said. 'Everybody, please carry on enjoying yourselves[6], and forget about it, would you[7]?' He forced yet another smile. 'I'm going to have another glass of wine, and I hope you'll all join me.'

Conversation broke out in scattered places[8], and gradually spread[9] until it filled the room with a continuous buzz[10], and the crisis was over[11]. It had been a bad mistake to tell Usher the news[12] here in the gallery at a reception: there was no doubt of that. Lampeth had made the decision at the end of a long, exciting day. In future he would go home early, or start work late, he resolved[13]. He was too old to push himself[14].

He found a glass of wine and drank it down quickly. It steadied his shaking knees[15], and he stopped sweating. God, how embarrassing. Bloody artists.

1. la tête haute
2. pour pouvoir suivre
3. ses grandes enjambées
4. en évitant le regard
5. Je vous prie de m'excuser pour...
6. continuez de vous amuser
7. si vous le voulez bien
8. Les conversations reprirent ici et là
9. se propagèrent peu à peu
10. d'un murmure permanent
11. terminée
12. d'avoir appris la nouvelle à Usher
13. décida-t-il
14. pour se surmener
15. Ses genoux s'arrêtèrent de trembler

Chapter Three

Peter Usher leaned his bicycle against the plate-glass window[1] of Dixon & Dixon's gallery in Bond Street. He took off his bicycle clips[2] and shook each leg in turn[3] to let the creases fall out[4] of his trousers. He checked his appearance in the glass[5]: his cheap chalk-stripe suit[6] looked a little crumpled[7], but the white shirt and wide tie and waistcoat[8] gave him a certain elegance. He was sweating under the clothes. The ride[9] from Clapham had been long and hot, but he could not afford tube fares[10].

He swallowed his pride[11], resolved again to be courteous, humble and good-tempered[12], and entered the gallery.

A pretty girl with spectacles and a mini-skirt[13] approached him[14] in the reception area. She probably makes more per week[15] than I do, Peter thought grimly[16] – then he reminded himself of his resolution[17], and quelled the thought[18].

The girl smiled pleasantly. 'Can I help you, sir?'

'I'd like to see Mr Dixon, if I may[19]. My name is Peter Usher.'

'Will you take a seat while I see whether Mr Dixon is in[20]?'

'Thank you.'

Peter sat back on a green leatherette[21] chair and watched the girl sit at her desk and pick up a telephone. He could see under the desk, between the drawer stacks[22], the girl's knees. She shifted[23] in her seat, her legs parted[24], and he looked at the smooth-

stockinged inside of her thigh[1]. He wondered if . . .
Don't be a fool[2], he told himself. She would expect
pricey cocktails[3], the best seats[4] at the theatre, Steak
Diane[5] and claret[6]. He could offer her an underground movie[7] at the Roundhouse[8], then back to her
place[9] with a two-litre bottle of Sainsbury's Yugo-
slav Riesling[10]. He would never get past those knees.
'Would you like to go through to the office?' the
girl said.

'I know the way,' Usher said as he got up. He went
through a door and along a carpeted corridor to another door. Inside was another secretary. All these
bloody secretaries, he thought: none of them could
exist without artists. This one was older, equally desirable[11], and even more remote[12]. She said: 'Mr Dixon is terribly busy this morning. If you'll sit down
for a few moments, I'll let you know when he's free.'

Peter sat down again, and tried not to stare at the
woman. He looked at the paintings on the walls:
water-colour landscapes[13] of no great distinction,
the kind of art that bored him. The secretary had
large breasts, in a pointed bra[14], under her loose,
thin sweater[15]. What if[16] she were to stand up and
slowly pull the sweater over her head . . . Oh, Christ,
shut up, brain. One day he would paint some of
these fantasies[17], to get them out of his system. Of
course, nobody would buy them. Peter would not
even want to keep them. But they might do him
some good.

He looked at his watch: Dixon was taking his time.
I could do pornographic drawings for dirty magazines[18] – I might make some money, too, that way.
But what a prostitution of the gift in these hands[19],
he thought.

The secretary picked up a telephone in response
to a soft buzz[20]. 'Thank you, sir,' she said, and

1. l'intérieur
de ses cuisses,
galbé par les bas

2. Ne sois pas
ridicule

3. des cocktails
hors de prix

4. les meilleures
places

5. [filet
de bœuf, servi
avec une sauce et
flambé]

6. du bordeaux

7. un film
underground

8. [ancien
entrepôt
converti en salle
de spectacle]

9. chez elle

10. du riesling
yougoslave de
chez Sainsbury

11. tout aussi
désirable

12. distante

13. des
aquarelles de
paysages

14. un soutien-
gorge pointu

15. un pull léger
et ample

16. Et si, tout à
coup,

17. certains de
ces fantasmes

18. des revues
cochonnes

19. quelle façon
de prostituer
mon talent

20. une sonnerie
discrète

put it down[1]. She stood up and came around[2] the desk. 'Would you like to go in,' she said to Usher. She opened the door for him.

Dixon stood up as Peter walked in[3]. He was a tall, spare man[4] with half-lens glasses[5] and the air of a general practitioner[6]. He shook hands without smiling, and briskly[7] asked Peter to sit down.

He leaned his elbows[8] on the antique desk and said: 'Well, what can I do for you?'

Peter had been rehearsing the speech[9] all the way up on his bicycle. He had no doubt that Dixon would take him on[10], but he would be careful not to offend the chap, anyway[11]. He said. 'I haven't been happy[12] with the way the Belgrave is handling me for some time. I wonder whether you would like to show my work[13].'

Dixon raised his eyebrows. 'That's a bit sudden, isn't it?'

'It may seem so, but as I say, it's been simmering for a while[14].'

'Fair enough.[15] Let's see, what have you done recently?'

Peter wondered briefly[16] whether Dixon had heard about the row[17] last night. If he had, he was not saying anything about it. Peter said: '*Brown Line* went for six hundred pounds a while ago[18], and *Two Boxes* sold for five hundred and fifty.' It sounded good, but in fact they were the only pictures he had sold in eighteen months[19].

'Fine,' Dixon said. 'Now what has been the trouble[20] at the Belgrave?'

'I'm not sure,' Peter replied truthfully[21]. 'I'm a painter, not a dealer. But they don't seem to be moving my work at all[22].'

'Hmm.' Dixon seemed to be thinking: playing hard to get[23], Peter thought. At last he said: 'Well, Mr Ush-

---

er, I'm afraid I don't think we can fit you into our roster[1]. A pity.'

Peter stared at him, flabbergasted[2]. 'What do you mean, can't fit me in? Two years ago every gallery in London wanted me!' He pushed his long hair back from his face. 'Christ! You can't turn me down![3]'

Dixon looked nervous, as if fearing the young painter's rage[4]. 'My view[5] is that you have been over-priced for some time,' he said curtly[6]. 'I think you would be as dissatisfied with us as you are with the Belgrave, because the problem is basically not with the gallery[7] but with your work. In time its value will rise again, but at present few of your canvases deserve to fetch more than[8] three hundred and twenty-five pounds. I'm sorry, but that's my decision.'

Usher became intense, almost pleading[9]. 'Listen, if you turn me down, I may have to start painting houses. Don't you see – I must have[10] a gallery!'

'You will survive, Mr Usher. In fact you'll do very well. In ten years' time[11] you will be England's top painter[12].'

'Then why won't you take me on?'

Dixon sighed impatiently. He found the conversation extremely distasteful[13]. 'We're not your sort of gallery[14] at the moment. As you know, we deal mainly in late nineteenth-century painting, and sculptures. We have only two living artists under contract to our galleries, and they are both well established. Furthermore, our style is not yours.[15]'

'What the hell does that mean?[16]'

Dixon stood up. 'Mr Usher, I have tried to turn you down politely, and I have tried to explain my position reasonably, without harsh words or undue bluntness[17] – more courtesy, I feel sure, than you would grant me. But you force me to be utterly frank[18]. Last night you created a terribly embarrass-

1. que nous puissions vous intégrer dans notre liste
2. sidéré
3. Vous ne pouvez pas refuser !
4. comme s'il craignait la fureur du jeune peintre
5. Personnellement, je pense que
6. sans ménagement
7. au fond, ce n'est pas un problème de galerie
8. qui puissent se vendre au-delà de
9. se fit véhément, presque suppliant
10. il me faut
11. D'ici dix ans
12. le plus grand peintre anglais
13. désagréable
14. le genre de galerie qu'il vous faut
15. En plus, notre style ne correspond pas au vôtre.
16. Mais que voulez-vous dire par là ?
17. en mesurant mes propos et en restant poli
18. totalement franc

ing scene[1] at the Belgrave. You insulted its owner and scandalized his guests. I do not want that kind of scene at Dixon's. And now I bid you good day[2].'

Peter stood up, his head thrust aggressively forward[3]. He started to speak, hesitated, then turned on his heel[4] and left.

He strode along the corridor, through the foyer[5], and out into the street. He climbed on to his bicycle and sat on the saddle[6], looking up at the windows above.

He shouted: 'And fuck you, too![7]' Then he cycled away.

He vented his rage[8] on the pedals, kicking down viciously[9] and building up speed. He ignored traffic lights, one-way signs[10], and bus lanes[11]. At junctions he swerved on to the pavement[12], scattering pedestrians[13], looking distinctly manic[14] with his hair flowing in the wind behind him, his long beard, and his business-man's suit.

After a while he found himself cycling along the Embankment near Victoria, his fury exhausted. It had been a mistake to get involved with the art establishment[15] in the first place, he decided. Dixon had been right: his style was not theirs. The prospect had been seductive at the time: a contract with one of the old-line[16], ultra-respectable galleries seemed to offer permanent security. It was a bad thing for a young painter. Perhaps it had affected his work.

He should have stuck with the fringe galleries[17], the young rebels; places like the Sixty-Nine, which had been a tremendous revolutionary force[18] for a couple of years before it went bust[19].

His subconscious was directing him to the King's Road, and he suddenly realized why. He had heard that Julian Black, a slight acquaintance[20] from art school days, was opening a new gallery to be called the Black Gallery. Julian was a bright spark[1]: iconoclastic, scornful[2] of art world tradition, passionately interested in painting, although a hopeless painter[3] himself.

Peter braked to a stop outside a shop front[4]. Its windows were daubed with whitewash[5], and a pile of planks lay on the pavement outside. A signwriter on a ladder[6] was painting the name above the place. So far[7] he had written: 'The Black Ga'.

Peter parked the bike. Julian would be ideal, he decided. He would be looking for painters, and he would be thrilled to pull in[8] someone as well known as Peter Usher.

The door was not locked, and Peter walked in over a paint-smeared tarpaulin[9]. The walls of the large room had been painted white, and an electrician was fixing spotlights to the ceiling[10]. At the far end a man was laying carpet over the concrete floor[11].

Peter saw Julian immediately. He stood just inside the entrance, talking to a woman whose face was vaguely familiar. He wore a black velvet suit[12] with a bow tie. His hair was earlobe length, neatly cut[13], and he was good-looking in a rather public-school sort of way[14].

He turned around as Peter entered, an expression of polite welcome on his face, as if he was about to say 'Can I help you?' His expression changed to recognition[15], and he said: 'God, Peter Usher! This is a surprise. Welcome to the Black Gallery!'

They shook hands. Peter said: 'You're looking prosperous.'[16]

'A necessary illusion.[17] But you're doing well[18] – my God, a house of your own[19], a wife and baby – you realize you ought to be starving in a garret[20]?' He laughed as he said it.

Peter jerked an enquiry[21] toward the woman.

1. un petit malin
2. qui méprisait
3. très mauvais peintre
4. pila devant la devanture d'une boutique
5. badigeonnées à la chaux
6. Sur une échelle, un peintre en lettres
7. Jusque-là,
8. il serait ravi de récupérer
9. une bâche tachée de peinture
10. installait des spots au plafond
11. posait de la moquette sur le sol en béton
12. costume
13. étaient bien coupés
14. avec un style très école privée
15. L'expression sur son visage changea dès qu'il le reconnut
16. Les affaires ont l'air de marcher.
17. Il faut bien faire illusion.
18. toi, tu t'en sors bien
19. tu as acheté une maison
20. tu devrais être en train de crever de faim dans une mansarde
21. jeta un regard interrogateur

'Ah, sorry,' Julian said. 'Meet[1] Samantha. You know the face.'

The woman said: 'Hi.'

'Of course!' Peter exclaimed. 'The actress![2] Delighted.[3]' He shook her hand. To Julian he said: 'Look, I wondered if you and I could talk business[4] for a minute.'

Julian looked puzzled and a little wary[5]. 'Sure,' he said.

'I must be off[6],' Samantha said. 'See you soon.'

Julian held the door for her, then came back and sat on a packing case[7]. 'Okay, old friend: shoot[8].'

'I've left the Belgrave,' Peter said. 'I'm looking around for a new place to hang my daubings[9]. I think this might be it. Remember how well we worked together organizing the Rag Ball[10]? I think we might be a good team again.'

Julian frowned and looked at the window. 'You haven't been selling well lately[11], Pete.'

Peter threw up his hands[12]. 'Oh, come on, Julian, you can't turn me down! I'd be a scoop for you.[13]'

Julian put his hands on Peter's shoulders. 'Let me explain something to you, old mate[14]. I had twenty thousand pounds to start this gallery. You know how much I've spent already? Nineteen thousand. You know how many pictures I've bought with that? None.'

'What's it all gone on[15]?'

'Advance rent[16], furniture, decoration, staff, deposits on this, deposits on that[17], publicity. This is a hard business to get into, Pete. Now if I were to take you on, I'd have to give you decent space[18] – not just because we're friends, but also because otherwise it would get around[19] that I was selling you short[20], and that would harm my reputation[21] – you know what an incestuous little circle this is[22].'

'I know.'

'But your work isn't selling. Pete, I can't afford to use precious wall space[1] for work I can't sell. In the first six months of this year four London galleries went bankrupt[2]. I could so easily go that way.'[3]

Peter nodded slowly. He felt no anger. Julian was not one of the fat parasites of the art world – he was at the bottom of the pile[4], along with the artists.

There was no more to be said. Peter walked slowly to the door. As he opened it Julian called out: 'I'm sorry.'

Peter nodded again, and walked out.

He sat on a stool[5] in the classroom at seven-thirty[6], while the pupils filed in[7]. He had not known, when he took on the job of teaching art classes[8] in the local polytechnic[9], how grateful he would one day be for the £20 a week it brought in. The teaching was a bore, and there was never more than one youngster in each class with even a glimmering of talent[10]; but the money paid the mortgage and the grocery bill[11], just.

He sat silent as they settled behind their easels[12], waiting for him to give the go-ahead or to begin a lecture. He had had a couple of drinks on the way: the expenditure of a few shillings[13] seemed trivial[14] compared with the disaster which had overtaken his career[15].

He was a successful teacher, he knew: the pupils liked his obvious enthusiasm and his blunt, sometimes cruel assessments[16] of their work. And he could improve[17] their work, even the ones with no talent; he could show them tricks[18] and point out technical faults[19], and he had a way of making them remember.

1. mon précieux espace mural

2. ont fait faillite

3. Cela pourrait très bien m'arriver.

4. il était au bas de l'échelle

5. tabouret

6. à dix-neuf heures trente

7. entraient les uns derrière les autres

8. pour enseigner l'art

9. à l'institut technologique du coin

10. ne serait-ce qu'une once de talent

11. les courses

12. leurs chevalets

13. ces quelques shillings dépensés

14. ne représentaient pas grand-chose

15. qui s'était abattu sur sa carrière

16. sa façon directe, parfois cruelle, d'évaluer

17. faire progresser

18. des astuces

19. signaler les défauts techniques

1. voulait passer
le diplôme des
beaux-arts

2. passe-temps

3. tout en
travaillant
comme employés
de banque

4. programmeurs
informatiques

5. hochements
de tête

6. le meilleur
conseil

7. Renoncez.

8. il se consacre
entièrement à
l'art

9. en
s'investissant
corps et âme
dans ses toiles

10. avec ironie

11. tout ce qui lui
importe vraiment

12. ceux qui
s'engraissent

13. les femmes de
la haute société,
les marchands

14. des
avantages
fiscaux

15. par ailleurs

16. [sweet
Fanny Adams]
que dalle

17. en l'espace de
quelques années

18. à discerner ce
qu'il voulait faire

19. chez les
brocanteurs

20. dans des
galeries miteuses

21. atteignent

Half of them wanted to go in for Fine Art qualifications[1], the fools. Somebody ought to tell them they were wasting their time – they should make painting their hobby[2], and enjoy it all their lives while working as bank clerks[3] and computer programmers[4].

Hell, somebody ought to tell them.

They were all here. He stood up.

'Tonight we are going to talk about the art world,' he said. 'I expect some of you hope to become part of that world before too long.' There were one or two nods[5] around the room.

'Well, for those who do, here's the best piece of advice[6] anyone can give you. Forget it.[7]

'Let me tell you about it. A couple of months ago eight paintings were sold in London for a total of four hundred thousand pounds. Two of those painters died in poverty. You know how it works? When an artist is alive, he dedicates himself to art[8], pouring his life's blood out on the canvas[9].' Peter nodded wryly[10]. 'Melodramatic, isn't it? But it's true. You see, all he really cares about[11] is painting. But the fat guys[12], the rich guys, the society women, the dealers[13], and the collectors looking for investments and tax losses[14] – they don't like his work. They want something safe and familiar, and besides[15], they know nothing – sweet FA[16] – about art. So they don't buy, and the painter dies young. Then, in a few years' time[17], one or two perceptive people begin to see what he was getting at[18], and they buy his pictures – from friends he gave them to, from junk shops[19], from flyblown art galleries[20] in Bournemouth and Watford. The price rises, and dealers start buying the pictures. Suddenly the artist becomes (a) fashionable and (b) a good investment. His paintings fetch[21] astronomical prices – fifty thousand, two hundred thousand, you name it. Who makes the money? The dealers, the shrewd investors[1], the people who had enough taste to buy the pictures before they became trendy[2]. And the auctioneers[3], and their staff, and the salesroom[4], and their secretaries. Everybody but the artist[5] – because he's dead. Meanwhile, today's young artists are struggling to keep body and soul together[6]. In the future, their pictures will sell for astronomical sums – but that's no good to them now.

'You might think the Government would take a cut[7] on these big art deals[8], and use it to build low-rent studios[9]. But no. The artist is the loser, always.

'Let me tell you about me. I was somewhat exceptional – my work started to sell well during my lifetime[10]. I took out a mortgage and fathered a child on the strength of it. I was England's up-and-coming painter[11]. But things went wrong. I was "overpriced", they say. I went out of fashion. My manners don't quite fit in with polite society. Suddenly, I'm desperately poor. I'm on the scrap heap.[12] Oh, I've still got enormous talent, they say. In ten years' time I'll be at the top. But meanwhile, I can starve, or dig ditches[13], or rob banks[14]. They don't care – you see—' He paused, and realized for the first time how long he had been speaking, and how engrossed[15] he had been in his own words. The classroom was completely silent in the presence of such fury[16], such passion, and such a naked confession[17].

'You see,' he said finally, 'the last thing they care about is the man who actually uses his God-given gift[18] to produce the miracle of a painting – the artist.'

He sat down on the stool then, and looked at the desk in front of him. It was an old school desk with initials carved in the woodwork[19], and ancient ink stains soaked[20] into its wood. He looked at the grain, noticing how it flowed like an op-art painting[21].

1. les investisseurs futés
2. avant qu'elles soient tendance
3. les commissaires-priseurs
4. la salle des ventes
5. Tout le monde, sauf l'artiste
6. pour joindre les deux bouts
7. prélèverait sa part
8. ces énormes transactions sur le marché de l'art
9. des studios d'artiste à loyer modéré
10. de mon vivant
11. le peintre anglais le plus prometteur
12. On m'a jeté aux ordures.
13. creuser des fossés
14. braquer des banques
15. absorbé
16. face à ce déchaînement
17. cette confession si intime
18. ce don qu'il a reçu de Dieu
19. avec des initiales gravées dans la menuiserie
20. et de vieilles taches d'encre incrustées
21. un tableau d'art optique

The pupils seemed to realize that the class was over. One by one they got up, put their things together[1], and left. In five minutes the room was empty but for Peter, who laid his head on the desk and closed his eyes.

It was dark when he got home to the small terraced house[2] in Clapham. It had been difficult to get a mortgage on the place, cheap as it was[3], because of its age. But they had managed it[4].

Peter had turned handyman[5] and created a studio out of the upper floor[6], knocking down internal walls[7] and making a skylight[8]. The three of them slept in the bedroom downstairs, leaving one living room and the kitchen, bathroom and toilet in an extension at the back.

He went into the kitchen and kissed Anne. 'I relieved my feelings[9] by shouting at the kids, I'm afraid,' he said.

'Never mind,' she smiled. 'Mad Mitch has come to cheer you up[10]. He's in the studio. I'm just making some sandwiches for us.'

Peter went up the stairs. Mad Mitch was Arthur Mitchell, who had studied with Peter at the Slade[11]. He had become a teacher, refusing to go into the risky, commercial business of being a full-time artist[12]. He shared Peter's utter contempt for[13] the art world and its pretensions.

He was looking at a recently finished canvas when Peter walked in.

'What do you think of it?' Peter said.

'Bad question,' Mitch replied. 'It invites me to pour out a load of bullshit[14] about movement, brushwork[15], design, and emotion. Better to ask whether I would hang it on my wall.'

---

1. rassemblèrent leurs affaires

2. maison mitoyenne

3. même si elle n'était pas chère

4. ils y étaient parvenus

5. était devenu bricoleur

6. converti l'étage supérieur en studio

7. en abattant les cloisons intérieures

8. puits de lumière

9. Je me suis défoulé

10. pour te changer les idées

11. [L'école d'art réputée située à Londres]

12. la précarité financière des artistes à plein temps

13. Comme Peter, il méprisait totalement

14. C'est une invitation à débiter un tas de conneries

15. les coups de pinceau

'Would you hang it on your wall?'

'No. It would clash with the three-piece suite[1].'

Peter laughed. 'Are you going to open that bottle of Scotch[2] you brought with you?'

'Sure. Let's have a wake.[3]'

'Anne told you?'

'She did. You've discovered for yourself what I warned you of[4] years ago. Still, there's nothing like finding out on your own account[5].'

'I'll say.[6]' Peter fetched two grubby glasses from a shelf[7], and Mitch poured whisky. They put on a Hendrix record[8], and listened to the fireworks from the guitar[9] in silence for a while. Anne brought cheese sandwiches, and the three of them proceeded to get drunk[10].

'The worst of it,' Mitch was saying, 'the kernel, as it were,[11] of the shit, as it is[12]—'

Peter and Anne laughed at the mixed metaphor. 'Go on,' Peter said.

'The fundamental piece of godawful bollocks[13], is the uniqueness of a work[14]. Very few paintings are unique in any meaningful sense[15]. Unless there's something very tricky about it – like the Mona Lisa smile, to take the outstanding example[16] – then it can be repeated[17].'

'Not exactly,' Peter put in.

'Exactly where it matters[18]. A few millimetres of space, a difference in colour which is only just noticeable[19] – these things don't matter with your average fifty-thousand-pound painting. My God, Manet didn't paint an exact replica of an ideal picture in his head – he just put the paint roughly[20] where he thought it ought to go. He just mixed the colour until it seemed about right[21].

'Take[22] the *Virgin of the Rocks*[23]. There's one in the Louvre, one in the National Gallery. Everybody

1. Cela n'irait pas du tout avec mon canapé et mes fauteuils
2. [whisky écossais]
3. Faisons une veillée
4. Tu as découvert tout seul ce dont je t'avais prévenu
5. par soi-même
6. Absolument.
7. deux verres crasseux sur une étagère
8. disque
9. le crépitement des notes de guitare
10. entreprirent de se saouler
11. Le fond, pour ainsi dire,
12. de la question, en fait
13. Le fondement de cette grande foutaise
14. le caractère unique d'une œuvre
15. véritablement
16. l'exemple le plus frappant
17. reproduit
18. ce qui compte
19. qu'on remarque à peine
20. grosso modo
21. à peu près correct
22. Si tu prends
23. [La Vierge aux rochers, L. de Vinci, 1486.]

1. l'un d'eux est un faux, mais lequel ?
2. C'est celui de la National Gallery, disent les Français
3. établissait avec certitude
4. Il faudrait presque autant de génie
5. le faire correctement
6. à l'origine
7. N'importe quoi ! s'exclama Mitch.
8. Donne-moi
9. une course de chefs-d'œuvre
10. Peter se leva d'un bond. Chiche !
11. gaspiller
12. accrocha avec des punaises les deux feuilles de papier
13. choisis un peintre
14. le Fossoyeur
15. À vos marques, prêts, partez
16. esquissa le contour
17. une pelle
18. représenta de l'herbe par petites touches
19. un bleu de travail
20. le visage ridé et las d'un vieux paysan
21. observait, médusée
22. prenaient forme

agrees that one of them is a fake – but which?[1] The Louvre's, say the London experts. The National Gallery's, say the French[2]. We'll never know – but who cares? You just have to look at them to see their greatness. Yet if somebody found out for certain[3] that one was a fake, nobody would go to see it any more. Bullshit.'

He drank from his glass, and poured more whisky. Anne said: 'I don't believe you. It would take almost as much genius[4] to copy a great painting, and get it right[5], as it would to paint it in the first place[6].'

'Rubbish!' Mitch exploded.[7] 'I'll prove it. Gimme[8] a canvas, and I'll paint you a Van Gogh in twenty minutes.'

'He's right,' Peter said. 'I could do it, too.'

'But not as fast as me,' said Mitch.

'Faster.'

'Right,' said Mitch. He got to his feet. 'We'll have a Masterpiece Race[9].'

Peter jumped up. 'You're on.[10] Now – two sheets of paper – we can't waste[11] canvas.'

Anne laughed. 'You're both mad.'

Mitch pinned the two bits of paper[12] on the wall while Peter got two palettes out.

Mitch said: 'Name a painter[13], Anne.'

'All right – Van Gogh.'

'Give us a name for the picture.'

'Umm – the Gravedigger[14].'

'Now say ready, steady, go[15].'

'Ready, steady, go.'

The two began painting furiously. Peter outlined[16] a man leaning on a shovel[17], dabbed in some grass[18] at his feet, and started to give the man overalls[19]. Mitch began with a face: the lined, weary face of an old peasant[20]. Anne watched with amazement[21] as the two pictures took shape[22].

They both took longer than twenty minutes. They became absorbed in their work, and at one point[1] Peter walked to the bookshelf[2] and opened a book at a colour plate[3].

Mitch's gravedigger was exerting himself[4], pressing the shovel into the hard earth[5] with his foot, his bulky, graceless body bent over[6]. He spent several minutes looking at the paper, adding touches, and looking again.

Peter began to paint something small in black at the bottom of his sheet. Suddenly Mitch yelled: 'Finished!'

Peter looked at Mitch's work. 'Swine,' he said.[7] Then he looked again. 'No, you haven't – no signature. Hahah!'

'Balls!'[8] Mitch bent over the picture and started to sign it. Peter finished his signature. Anne laughed at the pair of them.

They both stepped back at once.[9] 'I won!' they shouted in unison, and both burst out laughing.

Anne clapped her hands. 'Well,' she said. 'If we ever hit the breadline[10], that's one way you could make a crust[11].'

Peter was still laughing. 'That's an idea,' he roared[12]. He and Mitch looked at one another. Their smiles slowly, comically, collapsed[13], and they stared at the paintings on the wall.

Peter's voice was low, cold, and serious. 'Jesus Christ Almighty[14],' he said. 'That's an idea.[15]'

1. à un moment donné

2. l'étagère de livres

3. une planche couleur

4. s'épuisait à la tâche

5. enfonçant la pelle dans la terre dure

6. en arc-boutant son corps massif et peu gracieux

7. Fumier, dit-il

8. Merde !

9. reculèrent en même temps

10. si on sombre dans l'indigence

11. gagner votre croûte

12. dit-il, en éclatant de rire

13. s'estom-pèrent

14. Mais oui ! Bien sûr !

15. On pourrait faire ça.

Chapter Four

Julian Black was a little nervous as he walked into the entrance of the newspaper office[1]. He got nervous a lot these days[2]: over[3] the gallery, the money, Sarah, and his in-laws[4]. Which were really one and the same problem[5].

The marbled hall was rather grand[6], with a high ceiling, polished brass here and there[7], and frescoed walls[8]. Somehow he had expected a newspaper office to be scruffy[9] and busy[10], but this place looked like the lobby of a period brothel[11].

A gold-lettered signboard[12] beside the ironwork lift shaft[13] told visitors what was to be found on each floor. The building housed a morning and evening paper[14] as well as a clutch[15] of magazines and journals.

'Can I help you, sir?' Julian turned to see a uniformed commissionaire[16] at his shoulder.

'Perhaps,' Julian said. 'I'd like to see Mr Jack Best.'

'Would you fill in one of our forms[17], please?' Puzzled, Julian followed the man to a desk on one side of the foyer. He was handed[18] a little green slip of paper[19] with spaces for his name, the person he wanted to see, and his business[20]. This kind of screening process[21] was probably necessary, he thought charitably as he filled up the form with the gold Parker[22] in his pocket. They must get a lot of screwballs coming along[23] to a newspaper office.

It also made you feel rather privileged to be allowed to speak to the journalists, he thought. While he waited for the message to be taken to Best, he wondered about the wisdom[1] of coming in person. It might have been as well just to send out press releases[2]. He smoothed his hair and straightened his jacket[3] nervously.

There had been a time when nothing made him nervous. That was many years ago. He had been a champion schoolboy distance runner[4], head prefect[5], leader of the debating team[6]. It seemed he could do nothing but win[7]. Then he had taken up art. For the umpteenth time[8], he traced his troubles back to[9] that crazy, irrational decision. Since then[10] he had done nothing but lose. The only prize[11] he had won was Sarah, and she had turned out to be a phoney kind of victory[12]. Her and her gold Parkers, he thought. He realized he was clicking the button of the ballpoint[13] compulsively, and stuffed it back into his jacket pocket with an exasperated sigh. Her gold everything, and her Mercedes, and her gowns[14], and her bloody father.

A pair of scuffed, worn-down Hush Puppies[15] appeared on the marble steps and began to shuffle down[16]. Creaseless brown cavalry twills[17] followed, and a nicotine-stained[18] hand slid along the brass banister[19]. The man who came into sight was thin and looked rather impatient. He glanced at a green slip in his hand as he approached Julian.

'Mr Black?' he said.

Julian stuck out his hand. 'How do you do[20], Mr Best.'

Best put a hand to his face and brushed a long lock[21] of black hair off his face. 'What can I do for you?' he said.

Julian looked around. Clearly he was not going to be invited up to Best's office, or even asked to sit down. He ploughed on determinedly.[22]

1. il se demanda s'il avait bien fait
2. de diffuser des communiqués de presse
3. Il lissa ses cheveux et ajusta sa veste
4. À l'école, il avait été champion en course de fond
5. [élève] responsable de la discipline
6. le plus fort dans les ateliers de débat
7. que tout lui réussissait
8. énième fois
9. il situa l'origine de ses problèmes à
10. À partir de là
11. trophée
12. une fausse victoire
13. stylo à bille
14. robes
15. des Hush Puppies éculées et éraflées
16. à descendre d'un pas traînant
17. un pantalon sans pli, en serge marron
18. tachée de nicotine
19. rampe en cuivre
20. Ravi de vous connaître
21. repoussa une longue mèche
22. Il poursuivit, l'air déterminé.

'I'm opening a new gallery in the King's Road shortly[1],' he said. 'Naturally, as art critic of the *London Magazine* you'll be invited to the reception, but I wondered if I might have a chat with you about the aims[2] of the gallery.'

Best nodded noncommittally[3]. Julian paused, to give the man a chance to ask him up[4] to the office. Best remained[5] silent.

'Well,' Julian went on, 'the idea is not to get involved with[6] a particular school or artistic group[7], but to keep the walls free[8] for all kinds of fringe movements[9] – the kind of thing that's too way-out[10] for the existing galleries. Young artists, with radical new ideas.' Julian could see that Best was already getting bored.

'Look, let me buy you a drink, would you?'

Best looked at his watch. 'They're closed,' he said.

'Well, um, how about a cup of coffee?'

He looked at his watch again. 'Actually, I think the best plan would be for us to have a chat[11] when you actually open[12]. Why don't you send me that invitation, and a press release about yourself, and then we'll see if we can't get together[13] later on.'

'Oh. Well, all right then,' Julian said. He was nonplussed[14].

Best shook hands. 'Thanks for coming in,' he said.

'Sure.' Julian turned away and left.

He walked along the narrow street towards Fleet Street, wondering what he had done wrong[15]. Clearly he would have to think again about his plan of calling on[16] all the London art critics personally. He would write, perhaps, and send a little essay on the thinking[17] behind the Black Gallery. They would all come to the reception – there was free booze[18] at that, and they would know their pals[19] would be there.

God, he hoped they would come to the reception. What a disaster it would be if they did not turn up[1].

He could not understand how Best could be so blasé. It wasn't every week, or even every month, that a new art gallery opened in London. Of course, the critics had to go to a lot of shows, and most of them only had a few inches of space every week[2]. Still, you would think they would at least give the place a once over[3]. Maybe Best was a bad one. The worst[4], hopefully. He grinned, then shuddered, at his unconscious pun[5].

Nothing turned to gold any more[6]. He went back in his mind to the time when he had begun to lose his touch[7]. Deep in thought, he joined a bus queue[8] and stood at the kerb[9] with his arms folded[10].

He had been at art school, where he had found that everyone else was just as good as he at putting on that ultra-cool, throwaway hip style[11] which had stood him in such good stead[12] for the last couple of years at public school. All the art students knew about Muddy Waters and Allen Ginsberg, Kierkegaard and amphetamine, Vietnam and Chairman Mao. Worse[13], they could all paint – but Julian couldn't.

Suddenly he had neither style nor talent. Yet he persisted, and even passed exams[14]. It had done him little good. He had seen really talented people, like Peter Usher, go on to the Slade or wherever, while he had to scrabble around for jobs[15].

The bus queue moved convulsively, and Julian looked up to see the bus he wanted[16] waiting at the stop. He jumped on[17] and went upstairs.

He had actually been working when he met Sarah. An old school-friend who had gone into publishing[18] had offered him the job of illustrating a children's novel[19]. The money from the advance had

1. s'ils ne venaient pas

2. n'avaient droit qu'à un filet par semaine

3. viendraient au moins jeter un coup d'œil

4. Le pire

5. frémit à ce jeu de mots involontaire

6. Plus rien ne lui réussissait

7. il avait commencé à perdre la main

8. file d'attente

9. au bord du trottoir

10. les bras croisés

11. style branché et désinvolte

12. lui avait été si utile

13. Pire encore

14. avait même réussi ses examens

15. galérer pour trouver du travail

16. leva les yeux et vit son bus

17. Il monta

18. s'était lancé dans l'édition

19. un roman pour enfants

enabled him to kid[1] Sarah he had been a successful artist. By the time she found out the truth it was too late for her – and for her father.

The winning of Sarah[2] had made him think, for a little while, that he had got his old touch back[3]. Then it had turned sour[4]. Julian got off the bus, hoping she would not be at home.

The house was in Fulham, although Sarah insisted on calling it Chelsea. Her father had bought it, but Julian was forced to admit the old sod[5] had chosen well. It was small – three bedrooms, two recep. and a study[6] – but ultra-modern, all concrete and aluminium. Julian unlocked the front door[7] and went in, up the half-flight of stairs to the main living room[8].

Three of the walls were glass. Sadly, one enormous window looked on to[9] the road in front and another to the brick and pine end of a terraced row of houses[10]. But the rear window[11] had a view of the small garden, kept[12] neatly by a part-time gardener who spent most of his twenty hours per week smoking hand-rolled cigarettes and pruning the postage-stamp lawn[13]. And now the afternoon sun streamed in cheerfully[14], giving a pleasant glow[15] to the golden brown velvet of the upholstery[16].

One of the low, wide chairs was graced with the long body[17] of Sarah. Julian bent over and kissed her cheek perfunctorily[18].

'Good morning,' she said.

He resisted the temptation to look at his watch. It was about five o'clock, he knew, but she had only been up since midday[19].

He sat opposite her[20]. 'What are you doing?' he asked. She shrugged. There was a long cigarette in her right hand and a glass in her left[21]. She was doing nothing. Her capacity for doing nothing, hour after hour, never ceased to amaze[22] Julian.

She noticed his glance wander to her glass[1]. 'Have a drink?' she said.

'No.' He changed his mind. 'All right, I'll join you[2].'

'I'll get it.[3]' She stood up and walked over to[4] the bar. She seemed to be taking great care where she put her feet. When she poured his vodka it splashed up out of the glass on to the polished bar-top[5].

'How long have you been drinking?' he said.

'Oh, Christ,' she said. The blasphemy sounded foul coming from her[6]. She was a woman who knew how to make swear words count[7]. 'Don't start that.'

Julian suppressed[8] a sigh. 'Sorry,' he said. He took the drink from her hand and sipped it[9].

Sarah crossed one leg over the other, allowing her long robe to slip aside[10] and reveal a long, shapely calf[11]. Her beautiful legs were the first thing he had noticed[12] about her, he remembered. 'All the way up to her shoulders,' he had remarked coarsely[13] to a friend at that first party. And her height[14] had obsessed him ever since: she was a couple of inches taller than he[15] even without her outrageous platform shoes[16].

'How did it go?' she asked.

'Poorly[17]. I felt rather snubbed.'

'Oh dear. Poor Julian, always getting snubbed.'

'I thought we agreed not to begin hostilities.'

'Right.'

Julian resumed: 'I'm just going to send out press releases and hope the hacks will turn up[18]. It'll have to be a good do[19].'

'Why not?'

'Because of the money, that's why not. You know what I really ought to do?'

'Abandon the whole thing.[20]'

---

1. son regard qui s'attardait sur son verre
2. je t'accompagne
3. Je te le sers.
4. se dirigea vers
5. En servant la vodka, elle éclaboussa le bois ciré du bar
6. avait une résonance obscène dans sa bouche
7. qui savait donner du poids aux mots grossiers qu'elle prononçait
8. réprima
9. commença à le boire à petites gorgées
10. faisant glisser un pan du long déshabillé
11. un mollet long et bien galbé
12. qu'il avait remarqué
13. vulgairement
14. stature
15. elle le dépassait de cinq centimètres
16. très hautes chaussures à semelles compensées
17. Pas très bien
18. que les journaleux viendront
19. une réception réussie
20. Tout laisser tomber.

Julian ignored that. 'Give them all cheese sandwiches and draft bitter[1], then spend the money on paintings.'

'Haven't you bought enough?'

'I haven't bought *any*,' Julian said. 'Three artists have agreed to let me show their stuff on a commission basis[2] – if it sells, I get ten per cent[3]. What I really ought to do is buy the work outright[4]. Then if the artist catches on in a big way[5], I make a pile[6]. That's how these things work.'

There was a silence. Sarah offered no comment. Eventually Julian said: 'What I need is a couple of thousand more[7].'

'Are you going to ask Daddy?' There was a hint of scorn[8] in her voice.

'I can't face that.[9]' Julian slumped lower[10] in his chair and took a long pull[11] at his vodka and tonic. 'It's not just asking that hurts[12] – it's the certainty that he'll say no.'

'Quite rightly.[13] My God, I don't know what made him fork out[14] for your little adventure in the first place.'

Julian refused to rise to the bait[15]. 'Nor do I,' he said. He steeled himself[16] to say what he had to. 'Look, couldn't you scrape up[17] a few hundred?'

Her eyes flashed. 'You stupid little bastard[18],' she said. 'You touch my father for twenty thousand[19], you live in the house he bought, you eat the food I buy, and then you come to me for money! I have just about enough to live on[20], and you want to take that away. Christ.' She looked away from him in disgust[21].

But Julian had taken the plunge now[22] – he had nothing to lose. 'Look, you could sell something,' he pleaded. 'Your car would raise enough for me to set the gallery up perfectly. You hardly ever use it.[1] Or some of the jewellery you never wear[2].'

'You make me sick.' She looked back at him, and her lips flared in a sneer[3]. 'You can't earn money, you can't paint, you can't manage a bloody picture shop—'

'Shut up!' Julian was on his feet, his face white with anger. 'Stop it!' he shouted.

'You know what else you can't do[4], don't you,' she said. She pressed on remorselessly[5], turning the blade in the old wound[6] to see it bleed afresh[7]. 'You can't screw![8]' The last word was shouted, flung in his face like a blow[9]. She stood up in front of him, untied the cord[10] of her robe, and let the garment[11] slip from her shoulders to the floor. She took the weight of her breasts in her hands[12], caressing them with her splayed fingers[13]. She looked into his eyes.

'Could you do it to me now?' she said softly. 'Could you?'

Rage and frustration made him dumb[14]. His lips stretched bloodlessly[15] across his mouth in a rictus of humiliated fury.

She put one hand on her pubis and thrust her hips[16] forward at him. 'Try and do it, Julian,' she said in the same seductive tone. 'Try and get it up for me.'

His voice was half a whisper, half a sob[17]. 'You bitch[18],' he said. 'You bloody woman, you bitch.'

He rushed down the back stairs to the integral[19] garage, the memory of the row a twisting pain inside him[20]. He flicked the switch[21] that lifted the garage door, and got into Sarah's car. She was the kind of person who always left the keys in the ignition[22].

He had never borrowed her car before, hav ing been reluctant to ask; but now he took it

1. Tu ne t'en sers presque jamais.
2. certains des bijoux que tu ne portes jamais
3. un rictus déforma ses lèvres
4. de quoi tu es incapable aussi
5. insistait sans aucun remords,
6. remuant le couteau dans la plaie
7. pour la rouvrir
8. Tu es incapable de baiser !
9. asséné tel un coup de poing dans la figure
10. détacha la ceinture
11. vêtement
12. Elle soupesa ses seins à pleines mains
13. de ses doigts écartés
14. Il était muet de rage et de consternation
15. ses lèvres blêmes s'étirèrent
16. avança ses hanches
17. demi-sanglot
18. Espèce de salope
19. intégré
20. lui provoquant une douleur déchirante
21. Il appuya sur l'interrupteur
22. le contact

unrepentantly[1]. If she didn't like it, she would have to lump it[2].

'Cow[3],' he said aloud as he drove up the short, steep drive[4] and turned into the road. He headed south[5], towards Wimbledon. He ought to be used to these quarrels now: he was entitled to a degree of immunity. But the familiar jibes[6] seemed to hurt more with the passing of the years.

She was to blame as much as he, Julian thought. She seemed to take perverse pleasure in his impotence[7]. He had had a couple of girls[8] before Sarah. He had not been spectacular with them, he supposed: still, he had succeeded in doing what was expected[9]. It had some-thing to do with the very qualities[10] which had attracted him to Sarah – the perfection of her tall body, her immaculate aristocratic manners, her moneyed background[11].

But she could have put things right[12]. She knew what needed to be done, and it was quite within her power to do it[13]. Patience, kindness, and an un-hysterical attitude to sex would have cured him[14] years ago. But Sarah had given him indifference and contempt[15].

Perhaps she wanted him to be impotent. Maybe it protected her from sex; guarded her own short-comings[16]. Julian dismissed the thought. He was simply evading responsibility by transferring his blame to her[17].

He entered the drive of his father-in-law's[18] large house and stopped on the raked gravel[19] in front of the porch. A maid answered his ring at the bell.[20]

'Is Lord Cardwell at home?' he asked.

'No, Mr Black. He's at the golf club.'

'Thank you.' Julian got back into the car and drove off. He might have guessed the old boy[21] would be having a round of golf[22] on a fine evening like this.

He drove the Mercedes cautiously, not using its sprightly acceleration and cornering stability[1]. The car's power served only to remind him of his own ineffectiveness[2].

The golf club parking lot was crowded.[3] Julian left the car and went into the clubhouse. Sarah's father was not in the bar.

'Have you seen Lord Cardwell this evening?' he asked the bartender[4].

'Yes. He's having a round on his own. He'll be on the seventh or eighth[5] by now.'

Julian went out again and set off around the course[6]. He found Lord Cardwell putting on the ninth[7].

His father-in-law was a tall man with very thin white hair[8]. He wore a windbreaker and fawn slacks[9], and a canvas cap[10] covered most of his near-baldness[11].

'A nice evening,' Julian said.

'Isn't it. Well, now that you're here you can caddy for me[12].' Cardwell holed with a long putt, retrieved his ball[13], and walked on.

'How is the gallery coming along?' he asked as he prepared to tee off[14] on the tenth.

'Very well, in general,' Julian said. 'The redecoration is almost complete, and I'm working on the publicity at the moment.'

Cardwell flexed his legs, lined up the ball, and swung[15]. Julian walked beside him along the fairway[16]. 'However,' he continued, 'it's all costing an awful lot more[17] than I expected.'

'I see,' Cardwell said without interest.

'In order to ensure a good profit right from the start, I need to spend a couple of thousand buying paintings. But with the way money is flowing out[18] I shan't have it.'

1. sa reprise exceptionnelle et sa stabilité dans les virages

2. lui rappeler ses propres inaptitudes

3. Ｊe parking du club de golf était bondé.

4. barman

5. septième ou huitième trou

6. le parcours

7. en plein putting au neuvième trou

8. aux cheveux blancs très clairsemés

9. un coupe-vent, un pantalon couleur fauve

10. casquette en toile

11. sa quasi-calvitie

12. tu peux porter mes clubs de golf

13. fit le trou d'un long coup de putt, récupéra sa balle

14. prêt à jouer sa balle

15. fléchit les jambes, aligna la balle et fit un swing

16. [partie tondue/roulée du parcours entre le départ et le green]

17. bien plus

18. avec toutes les dépenses

'You will need to be very thrifty[1] at the start, then,' Cardwell said. 'It won't do you harm.'

Julian cursed inwardly[2]. This was the way he had feared the conversation might go. He said: 'Actually, I was wondering whether you might lay on[3] some extra cash. It would secure your investment[4].'

Cardwell found his ball and stood contemplating it[5]. 'You've got a lot to learn about business, Julian,' he said. 'I may be considered a rich man, but I can't lay on two thousand pounds at the drop of a hat[6]. I couldn't afford a three-piece suite[7] if I had to find the money tomorrow. But more important, you must learn how to go about raising capital[8]. You don't approach a man and say, "I'm a bit short[9]," could you lay on a few quid[10]." You tell him you're on to such a good thing[11] that you want to let him in on it[12].

'I'm afraid I can't let you have that extra cash. I put up the money in the first place against my better judgement[13] – however, that's in the past.

'Now let me tell you what I shall do. You want to buy some pictures. Now I'm a collector, not a dealer, but I know that the gallery owner's necessary talent[14] is the finding of good buys[15] in the picture market. Find some good buys, and I will give you that extra capital.'

He braced himself over his ball again[16] and prepared to swing.

Julian nodded soberly, trying hard[17] to keep his disappointment from showing on his face.

Cardwell swung powerfully[18], and watched the ball soar into the air[19] and land on the edge of the green[20]. He turned to Julian.

'I'll take those now,' he said, and slung[21] the golf bag on to his shoulder. 'You didn't come here to caddy for me, I know.' His tone became unbearably condescending.[1] 'Off you go[2], and remember what I said.'

'Sure,' Julian said. 'Cheerio.[3]' He turned away and walked back to the parking lot.

He sat in a traffic jam[4] at Wandsworth Bridge and wondered how to avoid Sarah for the rest of the evening.

He felt curiously free. He had done the unpleasant things he had been obliged to do, and was experiencing a sense of relief[5], despite the fact that he had achieved nothing[6]. He had not really expected Sarah or her father to cough up[7] – but he had been forced to try. He also felt quite irresponsible towards Sarah. He had rowed with her and pinched[8] her car. She would be furious with him, and there was nothing to be done for it.

He felt in his jacket pocket for his diary[9], to see whether there was anything he could go to. His hand found a slip of paper, and he brought it out.

The traffic shifted[10], and he moved the car off. He tried to read the piece of paper as he drove. It bore[11] the name Samantha Winacre, and an address in Islington.

He remembered. Samantha was an actress, and an acquaintance[12] of Sarah's. Julian had met her a couple of times. She had called at the gallery in passing the other day, and asked him to let her know what he was going to put on. The occasion came back to him[13]: that was when poor old Peter Usher had come in.

He found himself driving north, past the turning for home[14]. It would be rather pleasant to call on her[15]. She was very beautiful, and a talented, intelligent actress.

1. son ton condescendant devint insupportable

2. Allez, file

3. Salut.

4. Au volant, dans un embouteillage

5. il ressentait un certain soulagement

6. bien qu'il n'ait rien obtenu

7. crache au bassinet

8. lui avait piqué

9. Il chercha son agenda dans la poche de sa veste

10. La circulation reprit

11. Y était indiqué

12. une connaissance

13. lui revint à l'esprit

14. sans avoir tourné pour rentrer chez lui

15. de lui rendre visite

It was a poor idea[1] really. She would probably be surrounded by an entourage[2], or be out at show business parties all evening.

On the other hand[3], she did not seem the type for that sort of life[4]. All the same[5] he would need an excuse for calling. He tried to think of one.

He drove up Park Lane, negotiated Speakers' Corner[6], and went up the Edgware Road, eventually turning into Marylebone Road. He drove slightly faster now, looking forward to this slightly mad attempt to impose himself on[7] a film star. Marylebone Road became Euston Road, then he turned left at the Angel.

In a couple of minutes he was outside the house. It looked very ordinary[8]: no blasts of music[9], no noise of raucous laughter[10], no blaze of lights[11]. He decided to try his luck[12].

He left the car and knocked on the door. She came herself, her hair wrapped in a towel[13].

'Hello!' she said pleasantly.

'Our conversation was cut off[14] rather abruptly the other day,' Julian said. 'I was passing, and I wondered if I might buy you a drink[15].'

She smiled broadly. 'How delightfully spontaneous of you,' she laughed. 'I was just trying to figure out how to avoid spending[16] the evening in front of the telly. Come in.'

Chapter Five

Anita's shoes clattered cheerfully[1] on the pavement[2] as she hurried towards[3] Samantha Winacre's house. The sun was warm[4]; it was already 9:30. With luck, Sammy would still be in bed. Anita was supposed to start work[5] at nine o'clock, but she was often late, and Sammy rarely noticed[6].

She smoked a small cigarette as she walked, inhaling deeply[7], enjoying the taste of the tobacco[8] and the fresh morning air. This morning she had washed her long fair hair[9], taken her mother a cup of tea, fed her newest brother with a bottle[10], and got the rest of the children off to school[11]. She was not tired, for she was only eighteen; but in ten years' time she would look forty[12].

The new baby was her mother's sixth[13], not counting the ones that died and some miscarriages[14]. Did the old man not know about birth control, she wondered[15], or didn't he care? If he was my husband I'd make bloody sure he knew[16].

Gary knew all about taking precautions, but Anita wouldn't let him have it[17], not yet. Sammy thought she was old-fashioned, making a fellow wait. Perhaps she was, but she found it wasn't half so nice[18] unless you really liked each other[19]. Sammy talked a lot of nonsense[20], anyway.

Sammy's place was a terraced house with a basement[21], old but quite nicely done up[22]. Quite a lot of wealthy people had renovated old houses in this part of Islington, and the area was becoming quite

1. claquaient allègrement
2. le trottoir
3. tandis qu'elle se dirigeait d'un pas pressé vers
4. doux
5. était censée commencer
6. s'en apercevait rarement
7. en inhalant profondément
8. savourant le goût du tabac
9. ses longs cheveux blonds
10. donné le biberon à son plus jeune frère
11. aidé les autres enfants à se préparer pour aller à l'école
12. elle aurait l'air d'en avoir quarante
13. Ce nouveau-né était le sixième enfant de sa mère
14. quelques fausses-couches
15. À croire que son vieux ignorait tout de la contraception
16. tu m'étonnes que je le mettrais au courant
17. n'avait pas cédé
18. que c'était beaucoup mieux
19. si on s'aimait vraiment
20. disait beaucoup de bêtises
21. un sous-sol
22. refaite avec goût

1. était en train de devenir très chic
2. entra dans la maison
3. pour se maquiller
4. sauf pour sortir dans le West End
5. il y avait une publicité pour de la bière
6. de la vaisselle sale sur le bar
7. Elle retira ses chaussures de ville
8. sac en plastique
9. salon bas de plafond
10. D'étroites fenêtres haut perchées
11. filtraient la lumière
12. braqués sur des posters
13. petits tapis
14. sol en pavés de bois
15. les meubles de la pièce venaient de chez
16. mit de l'ordre
17. secoua les coussins pour les défroisser
18. jeta des fleurs qui commençaient à se faner
19. table d'appoint chromée
20. se demanda si elle avait le temps de faire la vaisselle

posh[1]. Anita let herself in[2] by the front door and closed it softly behind her.

She looked at her reflection in the hall mirror. There had been no time to put on make-up[3] today, but her round, pink face looked well without it. She never used much, unless she was going up West[4], of a Saturday night.

The mirror had an ad for ale[5] engraved in the glass, like something in a Pentonville Road pub. It meant you could never see the whole of your face in it, but Sammy said it was Art Deco. More nonsense.

She looked into the kitchen first. There were some dirty dishes on the breakfast bar[6], and a few bottles on the floor, but nothing much. Last night had not been a party night, thank God.

She stepped out of her street shoes[7], took a pair of moccasins from her carrier bag[8], and slipped them on. Then she went down to the basement.

The wide, low-ceilinged living room[9] took up the whole depth of the house. It was Anita's favourite room. Narrow windows high in the walls[10] at front and back let in a little light[11], but most of the illumination came from a battery of spotlights trained on posters[12], small pieces of abstract sculpture, and vases of flowers. Expensive scatter rugs[13] covered much of the block floor[14], and the room was furnished out of[15] Habitat.

Anita opened a window and tidied up[16] quickly. She emptied ashtrays into a bin, shook the creases out of cushions[17], and got rid of some flowers which were past their best[18]. She picked up two glasses from the chrome occasional table[19]; one smelled of whisky. Samantha drank vodka. Anita wondered whether the man was still here.

She went back to the kitchen and pondered whether she had time to wash up[20] before waking

Sammy. No, she decided; Sammy had an appointment[1] later in the morning. Still, she could probably clear the kitchen[2] while Sammy was drinking her tea. She put the kettle on[3].

The girl entered the bedroom[4] and pulled back the curtains, letting the sun pour through[5] like water from a bursting dam[6]. The bright light woke Samantha instantly. She lay still[7] for a moment, waiting for the last few cobwebs of sleep to dissolve in the awareness[8] of a new day. Then she sat up and smiled at the girl.

'Good morning, Anita.'

'Morning, Sammy.' The girl handed Samantha a cup of tea and sat down on the edge of the bed while she sipped it. Anita's accent had the broad twang[9] of a cockney[10] teenager, and her bustling, motherly manner about the house[11] made her seem older than she was.

'I've tidied downstairs and done the dusting[12],' she said. 'I thought I'd leave the washing until later. Are you going out?'

'Mmm.' Samantha finished her tea and put the cup down beside the bed. 'I've got a script conference.[13]' She threw the bedclothes aside[14] and got up, crossing the room to the bathroom. She got under the shower and washed herself quickly.

When she came out Anita was making the bed[15]. 'I got that script out for you,' she said. 'The one you was reading the other night.'

'Oh, thanks,' Samantha said gratefully[16]. 'I was wondering what I'd done with it[17].' With the huge bath towel wrapped around her[18], she went to the desk at the window and looked at the volume. 'Yes,

1. avait rendez-vous

2. ranger la cuisine

3. elle mit la bouilloire à chauffer

4. entra dans la chambre

5. et le soleil inonda la pièce

6. d'une digue rompue

7. Elle resta allongée sans bouger

8. pour finir d'émerger

9. le ton très nasillard

10. [Londonien né dans l'« East End »]

11. son attitude maternelle et affairée dans la maison

12. j'ai fait la poussière

13. J'ai une réunion pour discuter d'un scénario.

14. Elle repoussa les draps et les couvertures

15. faisait le lit

16. avec reconnaissance

17. ce que j'avais bien pu en faire

18. Enveloppée dans l'immense drap de bain

that's the one[1]. What on earth shall I do without you[2], girl?'

Anita busied herself about the room[3] and Samantha dried her urchin-cut hair[4]. She put on her bra[5] and panties[6] and sat in front of the mirror to make up her face. Anita was not as chatty[7] as usual this morning, and Samantha wondered why.

An idea struck her.[8] 'Have your A-level[9] results come yet?'

'Yeah. This morning.'

Samantha turned around. 'How did you do?'

'I passed,' the girl said flatly.[10]

'Good grades?[11]'

'Grade A in English.'

'That's terrific!' Samantha enthused.[12]

'Is it?'

Samantha stood up and took the girl's hands in her own. 'What is it[13], Anita? Why aren't you pleased?'

'It don't make no difference to anything, does it.[14] I can work in the bank for twenty pounds a week, or work in the Brassey's factory for twenty-five pounds. I could do that without A-levels.'

'But I thought you wanted to go to college[15].'

Anita turned away. 'That was just a silly thing[16] – a dream. I could no more go to college than fly to the moon. What'll you wear – the white Gatsby dress?' She opened the wardrobe[17] door.

Samantha went back to her mirror. 'Yes,' she said absently. 'Lots of girls go to college nowadays, you know.'

Anita laid the dress on the bed and put out white tights[18] and shoes. 'You know what it's like up my place[19], Sammy. The old man's in and out of work[20], no fault of his own. My mum can't earn much, and I'm the eldest, see[21]. I'll have to stop home[22] and work for a few years until the little ones[1] start bringing some money home. Actually—'

Samantha put down her lipstick[2] and looked past her own image in the mirror to[3] the young girl who stood behind her. 'What?'

'I was hoping you might keep me on[4].'

Samantha said nothing for a moment. She had employed Anita as a sort of maid-cum-housekeeper[5] during the girl's summer holidays. The two of them got on well[6], and Anita had turned out to be more than efficient[7]. But it had never occurred to Samantha[8] that the arrangement might become permanent.

She said: 'I think you ought to go to college.'

'Fair enough[9],' Anita replied. She picked up the teacup from the bedside table[10] and went out.

Samantha put the final touches to her face and dressed in jeans and denim shirt[11] before going downstairs. As she entered the kitchen Anita put a boiled egg and a rack of toast[12] on the small table. Samantha sat down to eat.

Anita poured two cups of coffee and sat down opposite her. Samantha ate in silence, then pushed her plate away and dropped a saccharine tablet[13] into the coffee. Anita took out a short filter-tipped cigarette[14] and lit it.

'Now listen,' Samantha said. 'If you must get a job, I'd be delighted for you to work for me. You're a terrific help. But you mustn't give up hope[15] of going to college.'

'There's no point in hoping. It's not on.[16']

'I'll tell you what I'm going to do. I'll employ you, and pay you the same as I'm paying you now[17]. You go to college in the term[18], and work for me in the holidays – and get the same money all the year round[19]. That way I don't lose you, you can help your mother, and you can study.'

1. les petits
2. rouge à lèvres
3. ignorant son reflet dans le miroir, regarda
4. que vous me gardериez
5. domestique et gouvernante à la fois
6. s'entendaient bien
7. s'était révélée plus qu'efficace
8. Samantha n'aurait jamais pensé
9. Très bien
10. table de chevet
11. chemise en jean
12. un œuf dur et un porte-toasts garni
13. Sucrette
14. cigarette filtre
15. renoncer à l'idée
16. Ça ne sert à rien d'espérer. C'est fichu.
17. je te verserai le même salaire que maintenant
18. pendant l'année universitaire
19. tout au long de l'année

1. les yeux
écarquillés
2. Vous êtes
tellement gentille
3. je ne dépense
presque rien
4. que je rends
service à
quelqu'un
5. sacré coup de
chance
6. Je vais
demander à
mon avocat de
rédiger
7. pour que tu
sois tranquille
8. Maintenant,
il faut que je file.
9. J'appelle un
taxi
10. légère
11. salaire
12. elle se sentit
étrangement
coupable
13. Ce n'était
pas normal
14. déductible
des impôts
15. une impo-
sante demeure
16. domestique
à plein temps
17. Elle ne
possédait
ni terres, ni
tableaux, ni
antiquités.
18. Elle se mit
à penser à cet
homme
19. Il avait été
assez décevant
20. tous ceux qui
débarquaient à
l'improviste
21. partaient du
principe

Anita looked at her wide-eyed[1]. 'You're ever so kind[2],' she said.

'No. I've got much more money than I deserve, and I hardly spend any of it[3]. Please say yes, Anita. I could feel I was doing somebody some good[4].'

'Mum would say it's charity.'

'You're eighteen now – you don't have to do what she says.'

'No.' The girl smiled. 'Thank you.' She stood up and impulsively kissed Samantha. There were tears in her eyes. 'What a bleedin' turn-up[5],' she said.

Samantha stood up, slightly embarrassed. 'I'll get my lawyer to draw up[6] some kind of thing to make it secure for you[7]. Now I must fly.[8]'

'I'll 'ring for a cab[9],' said Anita.

Samantha went upstairs to change. As she put on the flimsy[10] white dress which had cost more than Anita's wages[11] for two months, she felt oddly guilty[12]. It was wrong[13] that she should be able to change the course of a young girl's life with such a small gesture. The money it would cost would be negligible – and probably tax-deductible[14], she realized suddenly. It made no difference. What she had told Anita was true. Samantha could quite easily have lived in a stately home[15] in Surrey, or a villa in the South of France: she spent virtually nothing of her vast earnings. Anita was the only full-time servant[16] she had ever employed. She lived in this modest house in Islington. She had no car, no yacht. She owned no land, oil paintings or antiques.[17]

Her thoughts turned to the man[18] who had called last night – what was his name? Julian Black. He had been a bit of a disappointment[19]. In theory, anyone who called on her on the hop[20] had to be interesting: for everyone assumed[21] they would have to pass through a battery of security guards to get at her, and the duller sort of visitor[1] never bothered[2] to try.

Julian had been pleasant enough, and fascinating on his own subject, which was art. But it had not taken Samantha long to find out that he was unhappy with his wife[3] and worried about money[4]; and those two things seemed to sum up his character[5]. She had made it clear[6] she did not want to be seduced by him, and he had made no advances. They had enjoyed a couple of drinks and he had left.

She could have solved his problems as easily as she had solved Anita's. Perhaps she ought to have offered him money. He didn't seem to be asking for it, but it was clear he needed it.

Perhaps she ought to patronize artists[7]. But the art world was such a pretentious upper-class scene[8]. Money was spent with no clear idea of its value to real people: people like Anita and her family. No, art was not the solution to[9] Samantha's dilemma.

There was a ring at the door. She looked out of the window. The taxi was outside. She picked up her script and went down.

She sat back in the comfortable seat of the black cab[10] and flipped through[11] the script she was going to discuss with her agent and a film producer. It was called *Thirteenth Night*, which would not sell any cinema tickets[12]: but that was a detail. It was a reworking[13] of Shakespeare's *Twelfth Night*[14], but without the original dialogue. The plot made much of the homosexual innuendoes[15] in the play. Orsino was made to fall in love with Cesario[16] before the revelation that Cesario was a woman in man's clothes[17]; and Olivia was a latent lesbian[18]. Samantha would be cast as[19] Viola, of course.

The taxi stopped outside the Wardour Street office and Samantha got out, leaving the commission-

1. les visiteurs les plus barbants
2. ne se donnaient jamais la peine
3. pas heureux avec sa femme
4. qu'il avait des soucis d'argent
5. c'était ce qui l'avait marquée chez lui
6. Elle lui avait bien fait comprendre
7. parrainer des artistes
8. un milieu tellement aristocratique et prétentieux
9. ne pourrait résoudre
10. taxi [célèbres taxis noirs londoniens]
11. feuilleta
12. et ce n'était pas du tout vendeur
13. reprise
14. La Nuit des rois
15. L'intrigue s'appuyait sur des allusions à l'homosexualité
16. Orsino y tombait amoureux de Cesario
17. habillée en homme
18. était une lesbienne qui s'ignorait
19. aurait le rôle

aire to pay the driver. Doors were opened for her as she swept into the building, playing the role of a film star[1]. Joe Davies, her agent, met her and ushered her[2] into his office. She sat down and relaxed her public façade[3].

Joe closed the door. 'Sammy, I want you to meet Willy Ruskin.'

The tall man who had stood up as Samantha entered now offered his hand[4]. 'It's a real pleasure, Miss Winacre,' he said.

The two men were such opposites it was almost comical. Joe was short, overweight, and bald; Ruskin was tall, with thick dark hair over his ears[5], spectacles, and a pleasant American accent.

The men sat down and Joe lit a cigar. Ruskin offered Samantha a cigarette out of a slim case[6]; she declined.

Joe began: 'Sammy, I've explained to Willy here that we haven't come to a decision[7] on the script yet; we're still kicking it around[8].'

Ruskin nodded. 'I thought it would be nice for us to meet anyway. We can talk about any shortcomings you might think the script has[9]. And I'd naturally like to hear[10] any ideas of your own.'

Samantha nodded, collecting her thoughts[11]. 'I'm interested,' she said. 'It's a good idea, and the film is well written[12]. I found it quite funny. Why did you leave the songs out?[13]'

'The language is wrong[14] for the kind of film we have in mind,' Ruskin replied.

'Right. But you could write some new ones, and get a good rock composer to write tunes[15].'

'That's an idea,' Ruskin replied, looking at Samantha with a surprised respect in his eyes.

She went on: 'Why not turn the jester into a loony pop singer[16] – a kind of Keith Moon character[17].'

Joe interjected: 'Willy, that's a drummer with a British pop group[1]—'

'Yeah, I know,' Ruskin said. 'I like this idea. I'm going to get to work on it[2] right away.'

'Not so fast,' Samantha said. 'That's a detail. There's a much more serious problem with the film for me. It's a good comedy. Period.[3]'

'I'm sorry – why is that a problem?' Ruskin said. 'I'm not following you.'

'Me neither, Sammy,' Joe put in.

Samantha frowned. 'I'm afraid the thought isn't all that clear[4] in my own mind, either. It's just that the film doesn't say anything[5]. It's got no point to make[6], nothing to teach anyone, no fresh view[7] of life – you know the sort of thing.'

'Well, there is the thought that a woman can pose as a man[8] and do a man's job successfully,' Ruskin offered[9].

'That may have been subversive in the sixteenth century, but not any more.'

'And it has a relaxed kind of attitude to homosexuality[10] which might be thought educational.'

'No, it doesn't,' Samantha said forcefully[11]. 'Even television allows jokes[12] about homosexuals nowadays.'

Ruskin looked a little resentful[13]. 'To be candid[14], I don't see how the kind of thing you're looking for could be written into[15] a basic commercial comedy[16] like this.' He lit another cigarette.

Joe looked pained[17]. 'Sammy baby, this is a comedy. It's meant to make people laugh.[18] And you want to do a comedy, don't you?'

'Yes.' Samantha looked at Ruskin. 'I'm sorry to be so down on your script[19]. Let me think about it a little longer, will you?'

1. le batteur d'un groupe pop anglais
2. je vais y travailler
3. Sans plus.
4. que ce ne soit pas si évident
5. ne délivre aucun message
6. Il ne soulève aucune question
7. n'offre aucune nouvelle perspective
8. qu'une femme peut se faire passer pour un homme
9. suggéra Ruskin
10. il prône une attitude plutôt ouverte par rapport à l'homosexualité
11. avec véhémence
12. Même à la télévision, on plaisante
13. avait l'air quelque peu contrarié
14. Honnêtement
15. pourrait être transposé dans
16. comédie simple et grand public
17. prit un air contrit
18. Cela doit faire rire les gens.
19. d'être aussi sévère avec votre scénario

Joe said: 'Yeah, give us a few days, okay, Willy? You know I want Sammy to do it.'

'Sure,' Ruskin said. 'There's nobody better[1] than Miss Winacre for the part of Viola. But, you know, I have a good script and I want to get a film off the ground[2]. I'll have to start looking around for alternatives soon.'

'I'll tell you what, why don't we talk again in a week?' Joe said.

'Fine.[3]'

Samantha said: 'Joe, there are some other things I want to talk to you about.'

Ruskin got up. 'Thank you for your time[4], Miss Winacre.'

When he had left[5] Joe relit his cigar. 'Can you understand how I might feel pretty frustrated[6] about this, Sammy?'

'Yes, I can.'

'I mean[7], good scripts are few and far between[8]. To make life harder, you ask me to find you a comedy. Not just any comedy, but a modern one which will bring in the kids[9]. I find one, with a beautiful part[10] for you, and you complain[11] it doesn't have a message.'

She got up and went to the window, looking down upon the narrow Soho street[12]. A van[13] was parked, blocking the road and causing a traffic jam. A driver had got out and was abusing[14] the van driver, who ignored the imprecations and went about delivering[15] boxes of paper to an office.

'Don't talk as if[16] a message is something you only get in avant-garde off-Broadway plays[17],' she said. 'A film can have something to say and still be a commercial success[18].'

'Not often,' Joe said.

'*Who's Afraid of Virginia Woolf, In the Heat of the Night, The Detective, Last Tango in Paris.*'

'None of them[1] made as much money as *The Sting*.'

Samantha turned away from the window with an impatient jerk of her head[2]. 'Who the hell cares?[3] They were good films, and worth making[4].'

'I'll tell you who cares, Sammy. The producers, the writers[5], the cameramen, the second unit production team[6], the cinema owners, the usherettes[7], and the distributors.'

'Yeah,' she said wearily[8]. She came back to her chair and slumped in it[9]. 'Will you get the lawyer[10] to do something for me, Joe? I want a form of agreement drawn up[11]. There's a girl working for me as a maid. I'm going to put her through college[12]. The contract should say that I will pay her thirty pounds a week for three years on condition she studies[13] in the term and works for me in the vacation.'

'Sure.' He was scribbling the details on a pad[14] on his desk. 'That's a generous thing to do, Sammy.'

'Shit.' The expletive[15] raised Joe's eyebrows. Samantha said: 'She was going to stay at home and work in a factory, in order to help support the family. She's qualified[16] to go to university, but the family can't do without her earnings[17]. It's a scandal that there should be anyone like that while there are people earning what you and I earn. I've helped her, but what about the thousands of other kids in that position[18]?'

'You can't solve the world's problems all on your own, honey[19],' Joe said with a touch of complacency[20].

'Don't be so bloody condescending[21],' she snapped[22]. 'I'm a star – I ought to be able to tell people about this sort of thing. I should shout it from the rooftops[23] – it is not fair, this is not a just society. Why can't I make films that say that?'

1. Pas un seul
2. en secouant la tête avec impatience
3. On s'en fout !
4. qui valaient la peine d'être faits
5. les scénaristes
6. la deuxième équipe de production
7. ouvreuses
8. avec lassitude
9. s'y laissa tomber
10. Peux-tu demander à l'avocat
11. qu'il rédige une sorte de contrat
12. l'envoyer à l'université
13. sous réserve qu'elle étudie
14. Il griffonnait les éléments sur un bloc-notes
15. juron
16. Elle a les diplômes nécessaires
17. sans ses revenus
18. les milliers de gosses dans cette situation
19. à toi toute seule, ma chérie
20. une note de complaisance
21. Épargne-moi ta condescendance
22. dit-elle, d'un ton sec
23. le crier sur les toits

'All sorts of reasons – one being that you won't get them distributed[1]. We have to make happy films, or exciting films. We have to take people away[2] from their troubles for a few hours. Nobody wants to go to the pictures to see a film all about ordinary people having a hard time[3].'

'Maybe I shouldn't be an actress.'

'So what else are you going to do? Be a social worker[4], and find you can't really help people because you have too many cases to cope with[5], and anyway all they really need is money. Be a journalist, and find you have to say what the editor[6] thinks, not what you think. Write poetry[7] and be poor. Be a politician and compromise[8].'

'It's only because everyone is as cynical as you that nothing is ever done[9].'

Joe put his hands on Samantha's shoulders and squeezed affectionately[10]. 'Sammy, you're an idealist. You've stayed an idealist much longer than most of us. I respect you for it – I love you for it.'

'Ah, don't give me all that Jewish showbiz crap[11],' she said, but she smiled at him fondly[12]. 'All right, Joe, I'll think about this script some more. Now I have to go.'

'I'll get you a taxi.'

*

It was one of those cool, spacious Knightsbridge flats[13]. The wallpaper was a muted, anonymous design[14]; the upholstery was brocaded[15]; the occasional furniture antique. Open french windows[16] to the balcony let in the mild night air[17] and the distant roar of traffic[18]. It was elegant and boring.

So was the party. Samantha was there because the hostess was an old friend. They went shopping together, and sometimes visited each other for tea. But those occasional meetings had not revealed how far apart she and Mary had grown[1], Samantha reflected, since they had been in repertory[2] together.

Mary had married a businessman, and most of the people at the party seemed to be his friends. Some of the men wore dinner jackets[3], although the only food was canapés. They all made the most appalling kind of small talk.[4] The little group around Samantha was in an overextended discussion about an unremarkable group of prints[5] hanging on the wall.

Samantha smiled, to take the look of boredom off her face, and sipped champagne. It wasn't even very good wine. She nodded[6] at the man who was speaking. Walking corpses, the lot of them[7]. With one exception. Tom Copper stood out[8] like a city gent[9] in a steel band[10].

He was a big man, and looked about Samantha's age, except for the streaks of grey[11] in his dark hair. He wore a checked workman's shirt[12] and denim jeans with a leather belt[13]. His hands and feet were broad.

He caught her eye[14] across the room, and the heavy moustache stretched across his lips as he smiled. He murmured something to the couple he was with and moved away from them, towards Samantha.

She half-turned away from the group discussing the prints. Tom bent his head to her ear and said: 'I've come to rescue you from the art appreciation class[15].'

'Thanks. I needed it.' They had turned a little more now, so that although they were still close to the group, they no longer seemed part of it.

Tom said: 'I have the feeling you're the star guest.[16]' He offered her a long cigarette.

1. à quel point elle et Mary s'étaient éloignées

2. faisaient du théâtre de répertoire

3. des smokings

4. Tout le monde échangeait les pires banalités.

5. ensemble de lithographies quelconques

6. Elle hochait la tête

7. Tous des morts-vivants

8. se démarquait

9. un businessman de la City

10. L'orchestre à percussions métalliques, Caraïbes]

11. mèches grises

12. une chemise de trappeur à carreaux

13. ceinture en cuir

14. Il capta son regard

15. les amateurs d'art éclairés

16. J'ai l'impression que vous êtes l'invitée d'honneur.

1. *Ouais.*
2. *Et vous ?*
3. *Un représentant de la classe ouvrière.*
4. *avec ses initiales gravées*
5. *exagéra*
6. *J'suis un escroc, non ?*
7. *un accent pompeux*
8. *vers le buffet*
9. *une pointe de caviar au centre*
10. *Si c'est comme ça.*
11. *voyou*
12. *[l'école enseignant les bonnes manières]*
13. *les yeux de la tête*
14. *une fois par semaine*
15. *ça ne m'a pas servi à grand-chose*
16. *avocat*
17. *Il sortit un étui en fer-blanc de sa poche de pantalon*
18. *plaça deux gélules bleues dans le creux de sa main*
19. *que c'est de la drogue*
20. *Vous avez déjà pris du speed ?*
21. *Il glissa*

'Yeah.[1]' She bent to his lighter. 'So what does that make you?[2]'

'Token working-class representative.[3]'

'There's nothing working-class about that lighter.' It was slender, monogrammed[4], and seemed to be gold.

He broadened[5] his London accent: 'Wide boy, ain't I?[6]' Samantha laughed, and he switched to a plum-in-the-mouth accent[7] to say: 'More champagne, madam?'

They walked over to the buffet table[8], where he filled her glass and offered her a plate of small biscuits, each with a dab of caviar in its centre[9]. She shook her head.

'Ah, well.[10]' He put two in his mouth at once.

'How did you meet Mary?' Samantha asked curiously.

He grinned again. 'What you mean is, how does she come to be associated with a roughneck[11] like me? We both went to Madame Clair's Charm School[12] in Romford. It cost my mother blood, sweat and tears[13] to send me there once a week[14] – much good did it do me[15]. I could never be an actor.'

'What do you do?'

'Told you, didn't I? I'm a wide boy.'

'I don't believe you. I think you're an architect, or a solicitor[16], or something.'

He took a flat tin from his hip pocket[17], opened it, and palmed two blue capsules[18]. 'You don't believe these are drugs[19], either, do you?'

'No.'

'Ever done speed?[20]'

She shook her head again. 'Only hash.'

'You only need one, then.' He pressed[21] a capsule into her hand.

She watched as he swallowed three, washing them down with champagne. She slipped the blue oval into her mouth, took a large sip from her glass, and swallowed with difficulty. When she could no longer feel the capsule in her throat[1] she said: 'See? Nothing.'

'Give it a few minutes[2], you'll be taking your clothes off.'

She narrowed her eyes. 'Is that what you did it for?'

He did[3] his cockney accent again. 'I wasn't even there, Inspector[4].'

Samantha began to fidget[5], tapping her foot to nonexistent music. 'I bet you'd run a mile[6] if I did,' she said, and laughed loudly[7].

Tom gave a knowing smile[8]. 'Here it comes.[9]'

She felt suddenly full of energy. Her eyes widened[10] and a slight flush came to her cheeks[11]. 'I'm sick of this bloody party[12],' she said a little too loudly. 'I want to dance.'

Tom put his arm around her waist[13]. 'Let's go.'

1. gorge
2. Attendez quelques minutes
3. Il prit
4. Je plaide non coupable
5. à s'agiter
6. Je parie que vous partiriez en courant
7. se mit à rire très fort
8. afficha un sourire complice
9. Ça vient.
10. Ses yeux s'écarquillèrent
11. elle sentit que ses joues rougissaient légèrement
12. J'en ai marre de cette foutue soirée
13. mit son bras autour de sa taille

Part Two

The Landscape

'Mickey Mouse does not look very much like a real mouse, yet people do not write indignant letters to the papers about the length of his tail.'

E. H. GOMBRICH,
art historian

Chapter One

The train rolled slowly through the north of Italy. The brilliant sunshine had given way[1] to a heavy, chill cloud layer[2], and the scenery was misty and damp-smelling[3]. Factories and vineyards[4] alternated until they shimmered into a hazed blur[5].

Dee's elation[6] had dissipated gradually on the journey[7]. She did not yet have a find, she realized; only the smell of one[8]. Without the picture at the end of the trail, what she had found out was worth no more[9] than a footnote in a learned exegesis[10].

Her money was now running low.[11] She had never asked Mike for any; nor had she given him any reason to think she needed it. On the contrary, she had always given him the impression that her income[12] was rather higher than it really was. Now she regretted the mild deception[13].

She had enough to stay in Livorno for a few days, and for her fare home[14]. She turned away from the mundanity of cash[15] and lit a cigarette. In the clouds of smoke she daydreamed[16] what she would do if she found the lost Modigliani. It would be the explosive beginning to her doctoral thesis on the relationship between drugs and art.

On second thoughts[17], it might be worth rather more than that: it could make the centerpiece of an article[18] on how wrong everyone else was[19] about the greatest Italian painter of the twentieth century. There was bound to be enough of interest in the picture to start half-a-dozen academic disputes[20].

1. serait peut-être même connu sous le nom

2. cela la rendrait célèbre

3. assurée

4. un croquis au trait peu assuré

5. réalisé sous l'emprise

6. Ce ne pouvait être que

7. d'anti-conformiste et de précurseur

8. Et si c'était un abstrait

9. du début du siècle

10. pour savoir comment aller

11. le remettre triomphalement

12. dit-elle à haute voix

13. un petit bourg

14. sa rue principale et sa figure locale

15. des quais, des usines, une aciérie

16. seulement alors

17. station balnéaire

18. pour moderniser le port

19. mais tout avait été détruit sous les bombardements alliés

It might even become known as[1] the Sleign Modigliani – it would make her name[2]. Her career would be secure[3] for the rest of her life.

It might, of course, turn out to be a moderately good line drawing[4] like hundreds of others Modigliani had done. No, that was hardly possible: the picture had been given away as an example of work done under the influence[5] of hashish.

It had to be[6] something strange, heterodox, ahead of its time[7], revolutionary even. What if it were an abstract[8] – a turn-of-the-century[9] Jackson Pollock?

The art history world would be ringing up Miss Delia Sleign and collectively asking for directions[10] to Livorno. She would have to publish an article saying exactly where the work was to be found. Or she could carry it in triumph[11] to the town museum. Or to Rome. Or she could buy it and surprise the world by—

Yes, she could buy it. What a thought.

Then she could take it to London, and—

'My God,' she said aloud[12]. 'I could sell it.'

Livorno was a shock. Dee had been expecting a small market town[13], with half-a-dozen churches, a main street, and a local character[14] who knew everything about everyone who had lived here during the last hundred years. She found a town rather like Cardiff: docks, factories, a steelworks[15], and tourist attractions.

She realized belatedly[16] that the English name for Livorno was Leghorn – a major Mediterranean port and holiday resort[17]. Vague history-book memories floated back: Mussolini had spent millions modernizing the harbour[18], only to have it all destroyed by Allied bombers[19]; the town had something to do with the Medici[1]; there had been an earthquake[2] in the eighteenth century.

She found an inexpensive hotel; a high, white-washed[3] building in a terrace, with long, arched windows and no front garden. Her room was bare[4], clean and cool. She unpacked her suitcase, hanging the two summer dresses in a louvred cupboard[5]. She washed, put on jeans and sneakers[6], and went out into the town.

The mist had gone and the early evening was mild. The cloud layer was moving on, and the sinking sun was visible[7] behind its trailing edge[8] out across the sea. Old women in aprons[9], their straight grey hair pulled back and fastened at the nape of the neck[10], stood or sat in doorways[11], watching the world go by.

Nearer the town centre, handsome Italian boys paraded the pavements[12] in their tight-hipped, bell-bottomed jeans[13] and close-fitting shirts, their thick dark hair carefully combed[14]. One or two raised a speculative eyebrow at Dee, but none made a determined pass[15]. The boys were display items[16], she realized: to be seen rather than touched.

Dee strolled through the town aimlessly[17], killing time before dinner and wondering how to go about searching for the picture in this vast place. Clearly, anyone who knew of the picture's existence[18] could not know it was a Modigliani; and conversely[19], if anyone knew there was such a Modigliani they would not know where it was or how to find it.

She passed through[20] a series of fine, open squares, dotted with[21] statues of former kings[22] done in the good local marble. She found herself in the Piazza Vittorio, a wide avenue with central islands of trees and grass[23]. She sat down on a low wall to admire the Renaissance arcades.

1. Les Médicis
2. tremblement de terre
3. blanchi à la chaux
4. Sa chambre était simple
5. un placard à claire-voie
6. des tennis
7. on distinguait le soleil couchant
8. la traîne nuageuse
9. vêtues de tabliers
10. noués sur la nuque
11. sur le pas de leur porte
12. se pavanaient sur les trottoirs
13. jeans moulants à pattes d'éléphant
14. bien peignés
15. aucun ne lui fit des avances
16. étaient là pour se montrer
17. sans but précis
18. que ce tableau existait
19. et inversement
20. Elle traversa
21. jolies places ouvertes, parsemées de statues
22. anciens rois
23. des îlots de pelouse et d'arbres

It would take years to visit every house in the town and look at every old picture in attics[1] and junk shops. The field had to be narrowed down[2], even though that meant reducing the chances of success.

Ideas began to come at last. Dee got up and briskly walked back to the little hotel. She was beginning to feel hungry[3].

The proprietor and his family occupied the ground floor of the building. There was no one in the entrance hall[4] when Dee got back, so she knocked tentatively on the door[5] of the family's quarters[6]. Music and the sound of children filtered through, but there was no reply to her knock[7].

She pushed the door open and stepped into the room. It was a living room, with newish[8] furniture of appallingly bad taste[9]. A 1960s splayed-leg radio/record player[10] hummed in a corner. On the television a man's head soundlessly mouthed the news[11]. In the centre, on top of an orange nylon rug, a vaguely Swedish coffee table bore ashtrays, piled newspapers, and a paperback book.

A small child playing with a toy car[12] at her feet ignored her. She stepped over him[13]. The proprietor came through the far door. His stomach sagged hugely[14] over the narrow plastic belt of his blue trousers, and a cigarette bearing a precarious finger of ash[15] hung from the corner of his mouth. He looked at Dee enquiringly[16].

She spoke in fast, liquid Italian[17] 'I knocked, but there was no reply.'

The man's lips hardly moved as he said: 'What is it?[18]'

'I'd like to book a call[19] to Paris'

He moved to a bowlegged kidney-table[20] near the door and picked up the telephone. 'Tell me the number. I'll get it.'

Dee fished in her shirt pocket and took out[1] the scrap of paper[2] on which she had written the number at Mike's flat.

'Is there a particular person you want to speak to?' the proprietor asked. Dee shook her head. Mike was not likely to be back yet, but there was a chance that his char[3] would be in the flat – when they were away she dropped in whenever she felt like it[4].

The man took the cigarette out of his mouth and spoke a few sentences into the receiver.[5] He put the phone down and said: 'It will only be a few minutes. Would you like to sit down?'

Dee's calves ached slightly[6] after the walk. She sank gratefully into a tan leatherette armchair[7] that could have come from a furniture store in Lewisham[8].

The proprietor seemed to feel he should stay with her: either out of politeness, or for fear she might steal[9] one of the china ornaments on the mantelpiece[10]. He said: 'What brings you to Livorno – the sulphur springs[11]?'

She was not inclined[12] to tell him the whole story. 'I want to look at paintings,' she said.

'Ah.' He glanced around his walls. 'We have some fine work[13] here, don't you think?'

'Yes.' Dee suppressed a shudder[14]. The framed prints[15] around the room were mostly gloomy ecclesiastical pictures[16] of men with haloes[17]. 'Are there any art treasures in the cathedral?' she said, remembering one of her ideas.

He shook his head. 'The cathedral was bombed in the war.' He seemed a little embarrassed to mention the fact that his country had been at war with Dee's[18].

She changed the subject. 'I should like to visit Modigliani's birthplace[19]. Do you know where it is?'

---

1. fouilla dans la poche de sa chemise et en extirpa
2. bout de papier
3. femme de ménage
4. elle passait quand bon lui semblait
5. combiné
6. Les mollets de Dee étaient un peu endoloris
7. Elle s'affala avec soulagement dans un fauteuil en Skaï fauve
8. [banlieue du sud-est de Londres]
9. par politesse ou bien de peur qu'elle ne dérobe
10. bibelots en porcelaine sur le dessus de cheminée
11. les eaux thermales sulfureuses
12. n'avait pas envie
13. de belles œuvres
14. frisson
15. lithographies encadrées
16. des scènes religieuses lugubres
17. coiffés d'une auréole
18. son pays avait été en guerre contre celui de Dee
19. l'endroit où est né Modigliani

The man's wife appeared in the doorway and threw a long, aggressive sentence at him[1]. Her accent was too strong for Dee to follow. The man replied in an aggrieved tone[2], and the wife went away.

'Modigliani's birthplace?' Dee prompted.[3]

'I don't know,' he said. He took the cigarette out of his mouth again, and dropped it in the already-full ashtray. 'But we have some tourist guides for sale[4] – perhaps they would help?'

'Yes. I'd like one.'

The man left the room, and Dee watched the child, still playing his mysterious, absorbing game with the car. The wife walked through the room without looking at Dee. A moment later she walked back. She was not the most genial of hostesses[5], despite her husband's friendliness[6] – or perhaps because of it.

The telephone rang and Dee picked it up. 'Your Paris call,' the operator said.[7]

A moment later a woman said: ''Allo?'

Dee switched to French.[8] 'Oh, Claire, is Mike not back yet?'

'No.'

'Will you make a note of my number and get him to call[9]?' She read the number from the dial[10] then hung up[11].

The proprietor had returned meanwhile[12]. He handed her a small glossy booklet with curling edges[13]. Dee took some coins from her jeans pocket and paid him, wondering how many times the same book had been sold to guests who left it behind[14] in their rooms.

'I must help my wife to serve dinner,' the man said.

'I'll go in. Thank you.'

Dee crossed the hall to the dining room and sat down at a small circular table with a checked cloth[15].

Margin notes:

1. lui adressa une longue phrase de manière agressive

2. lui répondit sur un ton contrarié

3. lui rappela Dee

4. nous vendons des guides touristiques

5. une hôtesse très chaleureuse

6. gentillesse

7. Votre communication avec Paris, lui dit l'opératrice.

8. Dee enchaîna en français.

9. lui demander de me rappeler

10. sur le cadran

11. raccrocha

12. entre-temps

13. un livret en papier glacé tout corné

14. l'avait laissé en partant

15. une petite table ronde avec une nappe à carreaux

She glanced at the guidebook. 'The Lazaretto[1] of San Leopoldo is one of the finest of its kind[2] in Europe,' she read. She flicked a page. 'No visitor should miss seeing the famous Quattro Mori[3] bronze.' She flicked again. 'Modigliani lived first in the via Roma, and later at 10 via Leonardo Cambini.'

The proprietor came in with a dish of Angel's Hair soup[4], and Dee gave him a wide, happy smile.

*

The first priest was young, and his severely short haircut[5] made him look like a teenager[6]. His steel-rimmed[7] spectacles balanced on a thin, pointed nose[8], and he continually wiped his hands on his robes[9] with a nervous movement, as if drying the sweat from his palms[10]. He seemed edgy[11] in Dee's presence, as anyone who had taken a vow of chastity[12] was entitled to be; but he was eager to be helpful[13].

'We have many paintings here,' he said. 'There is a vault full of them in the crypt[14]. No one has looked at them for years.'

'Would it be all right for me to go down there?' she asked.

'Of course. I doubt if you'll find anything interesting.' As they stood talking in the aisle[15], the priest's eyes flickered[16] over Dee's shoulders, as if he was worried that someone would come in and see him chatting to[17] a young girl. 'Come with me,' he said.

He led her along the aisle to a door in the transept, and preceded her down a spiral staircase[18].

'The priest who was here around 1910 – was he interested in painting?'

---

1. [Lazaret, ancien établissement de quarantaine]
2. l'un des plus remarquables du genre
3. [monument dit « des Quatre Maures », XVIIᵉ s.]
4. une assiette de soupe au vermicelle
5. sa coupe de cheveux courte et sévère
6. un adolescent
7. à monture d'acier
8. tenaient en équilibre sur son nez fin et pointu
9. s'essuyait les mains sur sa soutane
10. les paumes de ses mains
11. Il avait l'air nerveux
12. ayant fait vœu de chasteté
13. ne demandait qu'à rendre service
14. Il y en a une salle pleine dans la crypte
15. dans l'allée centrale
16. le prêtre jeta un regard inquiet
17. bavarder avec
18. escalier en colimaçon

The man looked back up the stairs at Dee and then looked quickly away again. 'I've no idea,' he said. 'I am the third or fourth since that time[1].'

Dee waited at the foot of the stairs[2] while he lit a candle in a bracket on the wall[3]. Her clogs clattered on the flagstones[4] as she followed him, ducking her head through a low arch[5], into the vault.

'Here you are,' he said. He lit another candle. Dee looked around. There were about a hundred pictures stacked[6] on the floor and leaning against the walls of the little room. 'Well, I'll have to leave you to it[7],' he said.

'Thank you very much.' Dee watched him shuffle away[8], and then looked at the paintings, suppressing a sigh. She had conceived this idea the day before: she would go to the churches nearest[9] to Modigliani's two homes and enquire[10] whether they had any old paintings.

She had felt obliged to wear a shirt under her sleeveless[11] dress, in order to cover her arms – strict Catholics would not allow bare arms in church[12] – and she had got very hot walking the streets. But the crypt was deliciously cool.

She lifted the first painting from the top of a pile and held it up to the candle[13]. A thick layer of dust on the glass obscured the canvas underneath. She needed a duster[14].

She looked around for something suitable[15]. Of course, there would be nothing like that here. She did not have a handkerchief[16]. With a sigh, she hitched up her dress and took off her panties[17]. They would have to do.[18] Now she would have to be extra careful not to get the priest beneath her on the spiral staircase[19]. She giggled[20] softly to herself and wiped the dust off the painting.

It was a thoroughly mediocre oil of the martyrdom[1] of St Stephen. She put its age at about 120 years, but it was done in an older style. The ornate frame[2] would be worth more[3] than the work itself. The signature was illegible[4].

She put the painting down on the floor and picked up the next. It was less dusty but just as worthless.

She worked her way through[5] disciples, apostles[6], saints, martyrs, Holy Families[7], Last Suppers[8], Crucifixions, and dozens of dark-haired, black-eyed Christs. Her multicoloured bikini briefs[9] became black with ancient dust. She worked methodically, stacking the cleaned pictures together neatly, and working through one pile of dusty canvases before starting on the next.

It took her all morning, and there were no Modiglianis.

When the last frame was cleaned and stacked, Dee permitted herself one enormous sneeze[10]. The dusty air in front of her face swirled madly in the blow[11]. She snuffed[12] the candle and went up into the church.

The priest was not around[13], so she left a donation in the box and went out into the sunshine. She dropped her dusty panties in the nearest litter bin[14]: that would give the trash collectors[15] food for thought[16].

She consulted her street map and began to make her way towards the second house. Something was bothering her[17]; something she knew about Modigliani – his youth, or his parents, or something. She strained to bring the elusive thought to mind[18], but it was like chasing canned peaches around a dish[19]: the thought was too slippery to be grasped[20].

She passed a café and realized it was lunchtime. She went in and ordered a pizza and a glass of wine.

1. une huile vraiment médiocre du martyre
2. Le cadre très décoré
3. avait plus de valeur
4. illisible
5. Elle regarda un par un
6. des apôtres
7. des saintes Familles
8. des Cènes
9. slip
10. d'éternuer violemment
11. Le souffle fit tournoyer avec frénésie l'air chargé de poussière
12. éteignit
13. Elle ne vit pas le prêtre
14. la poubelle la plus proche
15. voilà qui donnerait aux éboueurs
16. de quoi gamberger
17. la dérangeait
18. Elle fit des efforts pour essayer de se rappeler
19. mais, comme des pêches en conserve lorsqu'elles fuient la cuillère dans une assiette,
20. le souvenir était insaisissable

As she ate[1] she wondered whether Mike would phone today.

She lingered over coffee[2] and a cigarette, reluctant to face another priest, another church, more dusty paintings. She was still shooting in the dark[3], she realized; her chances of finding the lost Modigliani were extremely slim. With a burst of determination[4], she stubbed[5] her cigarette and got up.

The second priest was older and unhelpful[6]. His grey eyebrows lifted a full inch[7] over his narrowed eyes as he said: 'Why do you want to look at paintings?'

'It's my profession,' Dee explained. 'I'm an art historian.' She tried a smile, but it seemed to make the man more resentful.

'A church is for worshippers[8], not tourists, you see,' he said. His courtesy was a thin veil.[9]

'I'll be very quiet.'

'Anyway[10], we have very little art here. Only what you see as you walk around[11].'

'Then I'll walk around, if I may[12].'

The priest nodded. 'Very well.' He stood in the nave[13] watching as Dee walked quickly around. There was very little to see[14]: one or two pictures in the small chapels. She came back to the west end[15] of the church, nodded to the priest[16], and left. Perhaps he suspected her[17] of wanting to steal.

She walked back to her hotel, feeling depressed. The sun was high and hot now, and the baking streets[18] were almost deserted. Mad dogs[19] and art historians, Dee thought. The private joke failed to cheer her up[20]. She had played her last card. The only possible way to carry on now was to quarter[21] the city and try every church.

---

1. En déjeunant,
2. prit son temps pour boire son café
3. avançait encore à l'aveuglette
4. Soudain très décidée
5. écrasa
6. était plus âgé et ne lui fut d'aucun secours
7. se haussèrent de plusieurs centimètres
8. les fidèles
9. Il était à peine poli.
10. De toute façon
11. en vous promenant dans l'église
12. si vous le permettez
13. Soit, dit-il, en restant planté dans la nef
14. Il n'y avait vraiment pas grand-chose à voir
15. extrémité ouest
16. fit un signe de la tête au prêtre
17. Peut-être la soupçonnait-il
18. sous la chaleur accablante, les rues
19. Mis à part des chiens enragés
20. ne la réconforta pas
21. de quadriller

She went up to her room and washed her hands and face to get rid[1] of the dust of the crypt. A siesta was the only sensible way to spend this part of the day[2]. She took off her clothes and lay on the narrow single bed.

When she closed her eyes the nagging feeling[3] of having forgotten something came back. She tried to remember everything she had learned about Modigliani; but it was not a lot. She drifted into a doze.[4]

As she slept the sun moved past the zenith[5] and shone powerfully in[6] through the open window, making the naked body perspire. She moved restlessly[7], her long face frowning[8] slightly from time to time. The blonde hair became disarrayed and stuck[9] to her cheeks.

She woke with a start[10] and sat up straight. Her head throbbed[11] from the heat of the sun, but she ignored it. She stared straight ahead of her[12] like someone who has just had[13] a revelation.

'I'm an idiot!' she exclaimed. 'He was a Jew![14]'

Dee liked the rabbi.[15] He was a refreshing change from the holy men who had only been able to react to her as forbidden fruit[16]. He had friendly brown eyes and grey streaks in his black beard[17]. He was interested in her search, and she found herself telling him the whole story.

'The old man in Paris said a priest, and so I assumed[18] it was a Catholic priest,' she was explaining. 'I had forgotten that the Modigliani family were Sephardic Jews[19], and quite orthodox.'

The rabbi smiled. 'Well, I know who the painting was given to[20]! My predecessor here was very eccentric, as rabbis go[21]. He was interested in all sorts

1. pour se débarrasser
2. Le plus raisonnable, à cette heure de la journée, c'était de faire la sieste
3. cette impression tenace
4. Elle s'assoupit peu à peu.
5. dépassa son zénith
6. pénétra de tout son éclat
7. Elle s'agita dans son sommeil
8. se crispant
9. Ses cheveux blonds, en bataille, collaient
10. Elle se réveilla en sursaut
11. Elle avait mal à la tête
12. Elle regarda droit devant elle
13. qui vient d'avoir
14. Mais il était juif !
15. Dee trouva le rabbin sympathique.
16. fruit défendu
17. sa barbe noire était grise par endroits
18. je suis partie du principe
19. juive séfarade
20. à qui le tableau a été donné
21. pour un rabbin

of things – scientific experiments[1], psychoanalysis[2], Communism. He's dead now, of course.'

'I don't suppose there were any paintings among his effects[3]?'

'I don't know. He became ill towards the end[4], and left the town. He went to live in a village called Poglio, which is on the Adriatic coast. Of course, I was very young then[5] – I don't remember him at all clearly[6]. But I believe he lived with a sister in Poglio for a couple of years before he died. If the painting still exists, she may have it.'

'She'll be dead.[7]'

He laughed. 'Of course. Oh dear – you've set yourself quite a task[8], young lady. Still, there may be descendants.'

Dee shook the man's hand. 'You've been very kind,' she said.

'My pleasure[9],' he said. He seemed to mean it.

Dee ignored her aching feet[10] as she walked back to the hotel again. She made plans: she would have to hire[11] a car and drive to this village. She decided she would leave in the morning[12].

She wanted to tell somebody; to spread the good news[13]. She remembered what she had done last time she felt this way[14]. She stopped at a shop and bought a postcard.

She wrote:

> Dear Sammy,
>
> This is the kind of holiday I always wanted! A real treasure hunt!![15] I'm off to Poglio[16] to find a lost Modigliani! ! !
>
> Love, D.

She found some change[17] in her pocket, bought a stamp[18], and posted the card. Then she realized that

KEN FOLLETT

she did not have enough money to hire a car and drive right across the country[1].

It was crazy: here she was[2] on the track of a painting which was worth anything from £50,000 to £100,000[3], and she couldn't afford to hire a car. It was painfully frustrating.[4]

Could she ask Mike for money? Hell, no, she could not lower herself.[5] Maybe she could drop a hint when he phoned[6]. If he phoned: his trips abroad did not follow tight schedules[7].

She ought to be able to raise money[8] some other way. Her mother? She was well off[9], but Dee had not invested any time with her for years. She had no right to ask the old woman for money. Uncle Charles?

But it would all take time. Dee was itching to get on the trail again[10].

As she walked up the narrow street to the hotel she saw a steel-blue[11] Mercedes coupé parked at the kerb[12]. The man leaning against it had a familiar head of black curls[13].

Dee broke into a run[14]. 'Mike!' she yelled happily.[15]

1. pour traverser le pays
2. elle était enfin
3. qui valait au bas mot entre 50 000 et 100 000 livres
4. C'était injuste et rageant.
5. Merde, elle ne pourrait jamais s'y abaisser.
6. faire une allusion, lorsqu'il appellerait
7. n'obéissaient pas à un calendrier très précis
8. trouver de l'argent
9. avait les moyens
10. trépignait, impatiente de poursuivre sa recherche
11. bleu métallisé
12. garée le long du trottoir
13. une chevelure de boucles noires qui lui était familière
14. se mit à courir
15. Mike ! cria-t-elle joyeusement

99

Chapter Two

James Whitewood parked his Volvo in the narrow Islington street and killed the engine[1]. He put a fresh packet of Players[2] and a box of matches[3] in one pocket, and a new notebook and two ballpoint pens[4] in the other. He felt the familiar tension[5]: would she be in a good mood[6]? Would she say something quotable[7]? His ulcer jabbed him, and he cursed[8]. He had done literally hundreds of star interviews[9]: this one would be no different[10].

He locked his car and knocked on Samantha Winacre's door. A plump[11] blonde girl answered.

'James Whitewood, *Evening Star*.'

'Please come in.'

He followed her into the hall. 'What's your name?'

'Anita. I just work here.'

'Nice to meet you, Anita.' He smiled pleasantly. It was always useful to be on good terms[12] with someone in a star's entourage.

She led him downstairs to the basement. 'Mr Whitewood, from the *Star*.'

'Hello, Jimmy!' Samantha was curled up[13] on a Habitat sofa, wearing jeans and a shirt. Her feet were bare. Cleo Laine[14] sang out of the freestanding[15] Bang & Olufsen stereo speakers opposite her.

'Sammy.' He crossed the room and shook her hand. 'Sit down, be comfortable[16]. What goes on in Fleet Street[17]?'

He dropped a newspaper in her lap[18] before sitting in an easy chair[19]. 'The big story of the day is

100

that Lord Cardwell is selling his art collection. Now you know why we call it the silly season[1].' He had a south London accent.

Anita said: 'Would you like a drink, Mr Whitewood?'

He looked up at her. 'I wouldn't mind[2] a glass of milk.' He patted his stomach.[3]

Anita went out. Samantha said: 'Is that ulcer still with you?'[4]

'It's like inflation. These days, you can only hope to make it ease off a little[5].' He gave a high-pitched laugh. 'Mind if I smoke?'[6]

He studied her as he opened the cigarette packet. She had always been thin[7], but now her face had a drawn look[8]. Her eyes seemed huge, and the effect had not been achieved with make-up[9]. She hugged herself with one arm[10] and smoked with the other. As he watched, she crushed a stub[11] in the full ashtray beside her and immediately lit a fresh cigarette[12].

Anita brought his glass of milk. 'A drink, Sammy?'

'Please.'

Jimmy glanced at his watch: it was 12:30 p.m.[13] He looked askance[14] at the size of the vodka and tonic Anita poured.

He said: 'Tell me, how is life in the film world?'

'I'm thinking of leaving it.[15]' She took the glass from Anita, and the maid left the room.

'Good God.' Jimmy took out his notebook and uncapped a pen[16]. 'Why?'

'There's not a lot to say, really. I feel films have given me all they can[17]. The work bores me[18], and the end result seems so trivial[19].'

'Is there any one particular thing which has triggered this off[20]?'

She smiled. 'You ask good questions, Jimmy. '

1. la période creuse
2. J'aimerais bien
3. Il se passa la main sur l'estomac.
4. Toujours votre ulcère ?
5. on ne peut que l'atténuer légèrement
6. Cela vous dérange si je fume ?
7. mince
8. elle avait les traits tirés
9. et ce n'était pas l'œuvre du maquillage
10. Un de ses bras étreignait son corps
11. elle écrasa un mégot
12. alluma une nouvelle cigarette
13. il était midi et demi
14. Il observa d'un œil désapprobateur
15. Je songe à arrêter le cinéma.
16. retira le capuchon d'un stylo
17. ne m'apportent plus rien
18. m'ennuie
19. le résultat n'a pas grand intérêt
20. qui a déclenché cela

He looked up expectantly[1], and saw that she was smiling, not at him, but at the doorway[2]. He turned, and saw a big man in jeans and a check shirt entering the room. The man nodded at Jimmy and sat beside[3] Samantha.

She said: 'Jimmy, I want you to meet Tom Copper, the man who has changed my life.'

Joe Davies pressed the winder of his Quantum wristwatch[4] and looked at the luminous red figures[5] which flickered alight on its black face[6]: 09:55. It was a good time to ring a London evening newspaper.

He picked up the phone and dialled[7]. After a long wait for the newspaper's switchboard[8], he asked for James Whitewood.

'Morning, Jim – Joe Davies.'

'A filthy morning[9], Joe. What load of old rubbish are you peddling[10] today?'

Joe could visualize the bad teeth exposed in[11] the grin on the writer's face: mock-hostile banter[12] was the game the two of them played to disguise the fact that each did his best to use the other. 'Nothing very interesting,' Joe said. 'A starlet landing a small part[13], is all. Just Leila D'Abo topping the bill[14] at the London Palladium.'

'That played-out old cow?[15] When's it coming off[16], Joe?'

Joe grinned, knowing he had won the game[17] this time. 'October 21, for one night.'

'Got it. By then she will just about be finished with that second-rate[18] film she's making at – where is it? Ealing Studios?[19]'

'Hollywood.'

'Yes. Now, who else is on the bill[20]?'

'Don't know. You'll have to ask the Palladium. You'll also have to ask them whether it's true that she'll be paid fifty thousand pounds for the appearance, because I'm not saying[1].'

'No, you're not.'

'Will that make a story for you?'

'I'll do my best for you[2], old son.'

Joe grinned again. If the story was good enough to get in the paper on merit[3], Whitewood would always pretend he was doing[4] the agent a personal favour. If the story was not good enough, the writer would say so.

Whitewood said: 'Now, have you given this to the opposition[5]?'

'Not yet.'

'Are you going to give us an edition start[6]?'

'As a personal favour to you, Jim – yes.' Joe leaned back in his leather-upholstered chair[7] with a feeling of triumph. Now the writer owed him[8] a favour. Joe had won on points.[9]

'Incidentally, what's up with your blue-eyed girl[10]?'

Joe sat forward suddenly[11]. Whitewood had a card up his sleeve[12] after all. Joe put a false nonchalance into his voice[13]. 'Which one?'

'Joe, how many of them did I interview this week? The malnourished[14] Miss Winacre, of course.'

Joe frowned[15] into the telephone. Damn Sammy. He was on the defensive now. 'I meant to ask you[16]: how did it go?'

'I got a great story – "Samantha Winacre retires[17]." Hasn't she told you?'

Christ, what had Sammy told the reporter? 'Between you and me, Jim, she's passing through a phase[18].'

1. parce que, moi, je ne t'ai rien dit

2. Comme c'est pour toi, je ferai de mon mieux

3. pour justifier un article dans le journal

4. faisait toujours croire qu'il accordait

5. à la concurrence

6. l'exclusivité

7. se laissa aller en arrière dans son fauteuil en cuir

8. lui devait

9. Joe avait marqué des points

10. Au fait, que se passe-t-il avec ta chouchou ?

11. se redressa d'un coup dans son fauteuil

12. avait un atout dans son jeu

13. adopta un ton faussement nonchalant

14. sous-alimentée

15. grimaça

16. Je voulais te demander

17. prend sa retraite

18. elle traverse une mauvaise passe

'An unfortunate one, it seems. If she's turning down[1] good scripts like *Thirteenth Night*, she must be pretty serious about retiring[2].'

'Do yourself a favour[3] – don't put that in your article. She'll change her mind.'

'Glad to hear it. I left it out anyway.'

'What line did you go on?[4]'

'Samantha Winacre says: "I'm in love." Okay?'

'Thank you, Jim. See you soon. Hey, just a minute – did she say who she's in love with?'

'The name is Tom Copper. I met him. Seems a sharp lad.[5] I should watch out[6] for your job.'

'Thanks again.'

'Bye.'

Joe put the phone down with a clatter[7]. He and Whitewood were even again[8] in the personal favour stakes: but that was the lesser misfortune[9]. Something was wrong[10] for Sammy to tell the reporter she was turning down a script without telling her agent.

He got up from his desk and walked to the window. He looked out at the usual traffic snarl-up[11]: cars were parked all the way along the double yellow lines[12]. Everybody thinks he's an exception, Joe thought. A warden[13] strolled along, ignoring the violations.

On the opposite pavement, an early-rising prostitute propositioned a middle-aged man[14] in a suit. Cases of cheap champagne were being carried into a strip club[15]. In the doorway of a closed cinema, an Oriental with short black hair and a loud suit[16] was selling a small packet of something to a haggard, unwashed girl whose hand trembled as she gave the man a note. Her gaunt face and butch haircut[17] made her look a little like Sammy. Oh, Christ, what to do about Sammy[18].

This guy was the key.[1] Joe went back to his desk and read the name he had scribbled on his pad: Tom Copper. If she's in love with him, she's under his influence. Therefore it is he who wants her to retire.

People hired[2] Joe to help them make money. People with talent: something Joe had never understood, except he knew he didn't have it. Just as Joe couldn't act to save his life[3], so his clients could not do business. He was there to read contracts, negotiate prices, advise on[4] publicity, find good scripts and good directors[5]: to guide naïve, talented people through the jungle of the show business world.

His duty to Sammy[6] was to help her make money. But that did not really answer the question.

The truth was, an agent was a whole lot more[7] than a businessman. In his time[8] Joe had been mother and father, lover, psychiatrist: he had provided a shoulder to cry on[9], bailed clients out of gaol, pulled strings[10] to get drugs charges[11] dropped, and acted as marriage guidance counsellor[12]. Helping the artist make money was a phrase which meant much more than it said out loud[13].

Protecting inexperienced people from the sharks[14] was a big part of it. Joe's world was full of sharks: film producers who would give an actor a part, make a pile out of the film, and leave the actor wondering where next month's rent was coming from; phoney gurus pushing quack religions[15], meditation, vegetarianism, mysticism or astrology who would milk a star[16] of half his income; screwball organizations[17] and semi-crooked businessmen[18] who would bamboozle[19] a star into supporting them, and then squeeze every ounce of available publicity out[20] of the association without regard[21] to the artist's image.

Joe was afraid Tom Copper was one of the sharks. It was all too fast; the guy had come from nowhere

1. La clé, c'était cet homme.
2. Les gens engageaient
3. Tout comme Joe n'aurait jamais pu être acteur
4. conseiller sur la publicité
5. metteurs en scène
6. Son devoir envers Sammy
7. beaucoup plus
8. À une époque
9. il avait été une oreille compatissante
10. tiré ses clients de prison, usé d'influence
11. qu'on abandonne les poursuites pour usage de stupéfiants
12. conseiller matrimonial
13. qu'il n'y paraissait
14. requins
15. les gourous véreux et leur charlatanisme religieux
16. capables d'extorquer à une vedette
17. des organismes bidon
18. des hommes d'affaires à moitié escrocs
19. embobinaient
20. exploitaient au maximum la publicité
21. sans se préoccuper

and suddenly he was running Sammy's life[1]. A husband she needed: a new agent she did not.

His decision was made. He leaned over his desk and pressed a buzzer[2]. The intercom hissed[3]: 'Yes, Mr Davies?'

'Come in right away, will you, Andy?'

He sipped his coffee while he waited, but it was cold. Andrew Fairholm – he pronounced it Fareham – was a smart lad[4]. He reminded Joe of himself. The son of a bit-part actor[5] and an unsuccessful concert pianist, he had realized at an early age[6] that he had no talent. Bitten with the show business bug[7] all the same, he had gone into management[8] and made a couple of second-rate rock groups into big earners[9]. About that time Joe had hired him as a personal assistant.

Andy entered without knocking and sat down in front of the desk. He was a good-looking youngster, with long, clean, brown hair, a wide-lapelled suit[10] and an open-necked shirt with a Mickey Mouse pattern[11]. He had been to university and cultivated a posh accent[12]. He was good for Joe's agency: gave it a slightly more modern image. His brain and youthful trendiness[13] complemented Joe's experience and renowned cunning[14].

'Trouble with Sammy Winacre, Andy,' Joe said. 'She's told a newspaper reporter that she's in love and she's giving up acting.'

Andy rolled his eyes up. 'I always said that chick was weird[15]. Who is the guy?'

'Name's Tom Copper.'

'Who the hell is he?'

'That's what I want to find out.' Joe ripped the sheet of paper[16] from his pad and handed it over[17]. 'Quick as you like.[18]'

Andy nodded and left. Joe relaxed slightly. He felt better with Andy working on the problem. For all his charm and fine manners[1], the lad had very sharp teeth[2].

*

It was a warm evening, with a summery smell in the still air[3]. The sunset over the rooftops[4] leaked blood into the high, sparse clouds[5]. Samantha turned away from the basement window and went to the cocktail cabinet[6].

Tom put a jazz record on the player[7] and sprawled on the sofa[8]. Samantha handed him a drink and curled up beside him. He put his large arm around her thin shoulders, and bent his head to kiss her. The doorbell rang.

'Ignore it[9],' he said, and kissed her mouth.

She closed her eyes and worked her lips against his[10]. Then she got up. 'I'd rather keep you in suspense.[11]'

It took her a few moments to recognize the short, velvet-suited man at the door. 'Julian!'

'Hello, Samantha. Am I bothering you?[12]'

'Not at all. Would you like to come in?'

He stepped inside the door, and she led him down the stairs. 'I won't keep you very long,' he said apologetically[13].

Julian looked a little embarrassed when he saw Tom on the sofa. Samantha said: 'Tom Copper, Julian Black.' Tom towered over Julian[14] as they shook hands. Samantha went to the bar. 'Whisky, isn't it?'

'Thank you.'

'Julian runs an art gallery[15],' Samantha said.

'That's a little premature. I'm opening one. What do you do, Tom?'

---

1. En dépit de son charme et de ses bonnes manières

2. ce garçon était redoutable

3. un parfum d'été flottait dans l'atmosphère figée

4. Au-dessus des toits, le soleil couchant

5. donnait aux rares nuages hauts une couleur rouge sang

6. bar à cocktail

7. un disque de jazz sur le tourne-disque

8. s'affala dans le canapé

9. N'y va pas

10. et l'embrassa à pleine bouche

11. Je préfère te tenir en haleine.

12. Est-ce que je vous dérange ?

13. d'un air confus

14. dominait Julian de toute sa hauteur

15. dirige une galerie d'art

1. par hasard
2. C'est pas dans mes cordes.
3. Disons que
4. toussa
5. qu'on se moquait de lui
6. en fait, c'est à propos de la galerie que je suis là.
7. s'installer confortablement
8. creux
9. quelqu'un qui présente bien
10. pour inaugurer le lieu
11. m'assurer que je n'ai pas d'autres engagements ce jour-là.
12. informations
13. Je ne vais pas vous déranger plus longtemps
14. si bien
15. Ravi de vous avoir rencontré
16. Il s'arrêta
17. posée
18. inutile de m'accompagner jusqu'en haut de l'escalier
19. son fichu magasin de tableaux

'You could call me a financier.'

Julian smiled. 'You wouldn't like to put some money into an art gallery, by any chance[1]?'

'Not my line.[2]'

'What is?'

'You might say[3] I take money from A and give it to B.'

Samantha coughed[4], and Julian had the feeling he was being laughed at[5]. He said: 'Actually, it's gallery business that brings me here.[6]' He took the drink Samantha handed him, and watched her settle snugly[7] in the crook[8] of Tom's arm. 'I'm looking for someone attractive[9] and interested to open the place[10]. Sarah suggested I ask you. Would you do it, as a favour to us?'

'I'd love to, but I'll have to make sure I'm not supposed to be somewhere else on the day[11]. Can I ring you later?'

'Sure.' Julian took a card out of his pocket. 'All the details[12] are on here.'

She took the card. 'Thanks.'

Julian swallowed his drink. 'I won't bother you any longer[13],' he said. He seemed slightly envious. 'You look so cosy[14]. Nice to meet you[15], Tom.'

He paused[16] at the door and looked at a postcard perched[17] on top of the thermostat on the wall. 'Who's been to Livorno?' he said.

'An old friend of mine.' Samantha got up. 'I must introduce you to her one day. She's just got a degree in art history. Look.' She took the postcard down, turned it over, and showed it to him. Julian read it.

'How fascinating,' he said. He handed the postcard back. 'Yes, I'd like to meet the lady. Well, don't bother to climb the stairs with me[18]. Goodbye.'

When he had gone Tom said: 'Why do you want to open his wretched picture shop[19] for him?'

'His wife's a friend. The Honourable[1] Sarah Luxter.'

'Which makes her the daughter of . . .?'

'Lord Cardwell.'

'The one who's selling his art collection?'

Samantha nodded. 'It's oil paint in the veins[2], you know.'

Tom did not smile. 'Now there's a caper.[3]'

The party was at the lifeless stage that parties go through[4] in the small hours[5] before they get their second wind[6]. The unrestrained drinkers[7] were getting sloppy[8] and disgusting and the restrained ones[9] were feeling the beginnings of their hangovers[10]. The guests stood around in clusters[11], concentrating on conversations which varied from intellectual to the comically incoherent.

The host was a film director just returned from the exile of television commercials[12]. His wife, a tall, thin woman whose long dress exposed most of what little bosom she had[13], welcomed Samantha and Tom and took them to the bar. A Filipino[14] barman whose eyes were glazing a little[15] poured whisky for Samantha and emptied two bottles of lager[16] into a pint glass for Tom. Samantha gave Tom a sharp look: he did not often drink beer, especially in the evening. She hoped he was not going to be aggressively working-class[17] all night.

The hostess made small talk[18]. Joe Davies detached himself from a group on the far side of the room and came over. The hostess, glad to be discharged[19], returned to her husband.

Joe said: 'Sammy, you have to meet Mr Ishi. He's tonight's star guest, and the reason we're all at the lousy party[20].'

'Who is he?'

1. [fille de lord]

2. La peinture à l'huile coule dans leurs veines.

3. Là, il y a un coup à faire.

4. avait atteint le point mort habituel

5. du petit matin

6. second souffle

7. Les buveurs invétérés

8. débraillés

9. ceux qui se tenaient encore

10. les prémices d'une gueule de bois

11. en troupeaux

12. après s'être exilé dans la pub télé

13. exhibait l'essentiel de sa petite poitrine

14. philippin

15. étaient un peu vitreux

16. bière

17. trop jouer le prolétaire

18. faisait la conversation

19. ravie d'être libérée

20. soirée pourrie

'A Japanese banker who is known to want to invest in the British film industry. He must be mad, which is why everyone's trying to get in with him[1]. Come on.' He took her arm, and with a nod to Tom, led her over to where a bald man with glasses was talking soberly to half-a-dozen attentive listeners.

Tom watched the introductions from the bar, then blew the froth off[2] the top of his lager and sank half of it[3]. The Filipino absent-mindedly[4] wiped the top of the bar with a cloth. He kept eyeing[5] Tom.

Tom said: 'Go on, take a drink – I won't tell on you[6].'

The barman flashed him a smile[7], grabbed a half-full glass from under the bar, and took a long swallow[8].

A woman's voice said: 'I wish[9] I had the courage to wear jeans – they're so much more comfortable.'

Tom turned to see a short girl in her twenties[10]. She was expensively dressed in imitation fifties clothes[11]: pointed, stiletto-heeled shoes[12], a tapered skirt[13], and a double-breasted jacket[14]. Her short hair was in a sweptback ducktail style[15] with a quiff[16] at the front.

He said: 'They're cheaper, too. And we don't have many cocktail parties in Islington.'

She opened her heavily shadowed eyes[17] wide. 'Is that where you live? I've heard that working-class men beat[18] their wives.'

'Jesus Christ,' Tom muttered[19].

The girl went on: 'I think that's awful – I mean, I couldn't stand[20] being beaten by a man. I mean, unless he was ever so nice[21]. Then I might like it. Do you think you would enjoy beating a woman? Me, for instance?'

'I've got better things to worry about,' Tom said. His contemptuous[22] tone seemed to be lost[23] on the girl. 'If you had some real problems to think about you wouldn't be making a fool of yourself[1] with me. Privilege breeds boredom[2], and boredom breeds empty people like you.'

He had needled the girl at last.[3] 'If that's how you feel, maybe you should choke on your privileged beer[4]. What are you doing here, anyway?'

'That's what I'm wondering.' He drained his glass[5] and stood up. 'Crazy conversations like this I don't need.'

He looked around for Sammy, but he heard her voice before he saw her. She was shouting at Joe Davies. In a second everyone was watching.

Her face was red, and she was more angry than Tom had ever seen her. 'How dare you investigate[6] my friends,' she yelled. 'You're not my guardian angel, you're my lousy fucking agent. You used to be my agent, because you're fired[7], Joe Davies.' She slapped the man's face once[8], hard, and turned on her heel[9].

The agent purpled in humiliation.[10] He stepped after Samantha with a raised fist[11]. Two long strides took Tom across the room[12]. He pushed Joe, gently but firmly, so that the agent rocked back on his heels. Then Tom turned and followed Samantha out of the room.

Outside on the pavement, she broke into a run. 'Sammy!' Tom called. He ran after her. When he caught up with her, he gripped her arm[13] and stopped her.

'What is this all about?' he asked.

She looked up at him, confusion and anger in her eyes. 'Joe had you investigated[14],' she said. 'He said you had a wife, four children, and a police record[15].'

'Oh.' He looked piercingly into her eyes.[16] 'So what do you think?'

---

1. vous ridiculiser

2. Les privilèges engendrent l'ennui

3. Il avait enfin réussi à mettre la fille en rogne.

4. vous étouffer avec votre bière de riche

5. vida son verre d'un trait

6. Comment oses-tu enquêter sur

7. tu es viré

8. Elle lui asséna une gifle

9. tourna les talons

10. Humilié, l'agent rougit.

11. Il commença à suivre Samantha, le poing levé

12. En deux grands pas, Tom traversa la pièce

13. Lorsqu'il la rattrapa, il lui saisit le bras

14. a fait enquêter sur toi

15. casier judiciaire

16. Il lui jeta un regard perçant

'How the hell do I know what to think?'

'I have a broken marriage[1], and the divorce isn't through yet[2]. Ten years ago I forged a cheque[3]. Does that make any difference to anything?'

She stared at him for a moment. Then she buried her head in his shoulder. 'No, Tom, no.'

He held her still in his arms[4] for a long moment. Then he said: 'It was a lousy party, anyway. Let's get a cab.'

They walked up to Park Lane and found a taxi outside one of the hotels. The driver took them along Piccadilly, the Strand, and Fleet Street. Tom got him to stop at a newsstand[5] where early editions[6] of the morning papers were on sale.

It was getting light[7] as they drove under Holborn Viaduct. 'Look at this,' Tom said. 'Lord Cardwell's paintings are expected to raise a million pounds.' He folded the paper and looked out of the window. 'Do you know how he got those pictures?'

'Tell me.'

'In the seventeenth century sailors died[8] to bring him gold from South America. In the eighteenth, farmers starved[9] to pay his rents. In the nineteenth, children died in factories and urban slums[10] to maximize his profits[11]. In this century he went into banking to help other people do what he had been doing for three hundred years – getting rich on poor men's backs[12]. Christ, a million pounds could build a nice little housing estate[13] in Islington.'

'What's to be done?' Sammy said disconsolately[14].

'Beats me.[15]'

'If the people won't take their money from him[16], we'll have to[17].'

'Oh yes?'

'Tom, be serious! Why not?'

He put his arm around her. 'Sure, why not. We'll steal[1] his paintings, sell them for a million quid, and build a housing estate. We'll sort out the details in the morning.[2] Kiss me.'

She lifted her mouth to his, and broke away quickly[3] 'I mean it[4], Tom.'

He looked at her face for a moment. 'Stone the crows[5], I think you do,' he said.

1. *Nous lui volerons*

2. *Nous réglerons les détails demain matin.*

3. *se dégagea brusquement*

4. *Je suis sérieuse*

5. *Mince alors*

Chapter Three

Julian lay awake[1]. The late August[2] night was unpleasantly warm[3]. The bedroom windows were open, and he had thrown the duvet off the bed[4], but he was still sweating. Sarah lay with her back to him on the far side of the wide bed[5], her legs spread in a striding position[6]. Her body gleamed palely[7] in the weak dawn light[8], and the shadowy cleft of her buttocks[9] was a mocking invitation[10]. She did not stir[11] when he got out of bed.

He took a pair of underpants from a drawer[12] and slipped into them. Closing the bedroom door softly[13] behind him, he went across the hall, down a half-flight of stairs, and through the living room to the kitchen. He filled the electric kettle[14] and plugged it in.

The words on the postcard which he had read the previous night in Samantha's living room were repeated again and again[15] inside his head, like a pop tune which refuses to be forgotten. 'I'm off to Poglio to find a lost Modigliani.' The message had burned its acid way[16] into his brain. It was that, more than the heat, which had kept him awake[17] ever since.

He had to go after[18] the lost Modigliani. It would be exactly what he needed – a real find[19]. It would establish his reputation as a dealer and attract flocks[20] of people to the Black Gallery. It was not in line with[21] gallery policy, but that did not matter.

Julian put a teabag into a mug and poured boiling water into it. He poked[22] disconsolately at the floating bag, submerging it with a spoon and watching it rise again[1] to the surface. The Modigliani was his golden opportunity[2], and he could see no way to snatch at it[3].

If he could find the picture, Lord Cardwell would put up the money to buy it. Sarah's father had promised that, and the old fool[4] could be trusted to keep his word[5]. But he would not fork out a penny[6] on the basis of a postcard from a scatty girl[7]. And Julian did not have the money to go to Italy.

The tea had turned a thick brown colour, and a hard-water scum[8] was forming on the surface. He took it over to the breakfast bar and sat on a high stool[9]. He looked around the kitchen, at the dishwasher[10], the split-level cooker[11] that was only used for boiling eggs, the washing machine, the freezer[12], and the host of smaller electric toys[13]. It was maddening[14] to be near so much wealth and unable to use it.

How much would he need? Air fare[15], hotel bills, perhaps a little bribery[16] . . . Everything depended upon how long it took him to catch up with the woman who signed herself D. A few hundred pounds – perhaps a thousand. He had to have the money.

He turned possibilities over in his mind as he sipped his tea. He could steal some of Sarah's jewellery and pawn it[17]. That might get him in trouble with the police. Did pawnbrokers demand proof of ownership[18]? Probably the good ones did. No, that was out of his field[19]. Forging one of her cheques[20] was more his style. But she would find out about that even sooner. And in both cases, it would be too risky to raise the kind of amount he needed.

1. avec une cuillère et le regardait remonter
2. lui offrait une opportunité en or
3. il ne voyait pas comment la saisir
4. ce vieux fou
5. pour tenir parole
6. il n'avancerait pas un centime
7. une écervelée
8. une pellicule de calcaire
9. tabouret haut
10. lave-vaisselle
11. [appareil de cuisson à éléments séparés]
12. congélateur
13. la foule de gadgets électriques plus petits
14. Cela le rendait fou
15. Le billet d'avion
16. un petit bakchich
17. les mettre en gage
18. Les prêteurs sur gage exigeaient-ils des titres de propriété ?
19. il n'était pas en mesure de faire cela
20. Imiter la signature de Sarah sur un chèque

He would have to find something she would not miss[1]. Something easily negotiable and worth a lot of money.

He could drive to Italy, he realized. He had looked up Poglio in the gazetteer[2] – it was on the Adriatic, in Northern Italy. He could sleep in the car.

But then he would find it difficult to look smart[3] if any careful negotiations were required[4]. And he would still need money for petrol, and meals[5], and bribes.

He could *tell* her he was driving to Italy, and then sell the car. Then she would discover his deception[6] as soon as he returned – just when he wanted her father to fork out. So, he could say the car had been stolen.

That was it.[7] He could say the car had been stolen – and sell it. She would want to notify the police[8], and the insurance company. But he could tell her he had dealt with all that[9].

Then there would have to be a delay[10], while the police were supposedly looking for it[11]. The insurance company could take months to fork out. By the time[12] Sarah realized it was all a deception, Julian's reputation would be established.

He was determined to give it a try[13]. He would go out and find a suitable garage[14]. He looked at his wristwatch. It was 8:30. He went back to the bedroom to put on his clothes.

He found the log-book[15] in a drawer in the kitchen, and the car keys where he had left them last night.

He ought to do something to make it all look convincing[16]. He found a sheet of paper and a blunt pencil[17], and wrote a note[18] to Sarah. 'Have taken the car. Will be out all day. Business. J.'

He left the note next to[1] the coffeepot in the kitchen, and went down to the garage.

It took him more than an hour to get through[2] the West End and the City and along the Mile End Road to Stratford. Traffic was heavy[3] and the road was hopelessly inadequate. When he reached Leytonstone High Road he found a rash of used car lots[4]: in shop fronts, on bomb sites[5], at gas stations[6], spilling on to the pavements[7].

He chose a largish one[8] on a corner. There was a young-looking Jaguar out front, and plenty of late-model quality cars[9] in the yard at the side. Julian drove in.

A middle-aged man was washing the windscreen[10] of a big Ford. He wore a leather hat and a short coat open at the front. He walked over to Julian carrying his rag and bucket of water[11].

'You're an early bird[12],' he said pleasantly. He had a heavy East End accent.

Julian said: 'Is the boss[13] around?'

The man's manner chilled perceptibly.[14] 'Speaking[15],' he said.

Julian indicated the car with a wave of his hand[16]. 'What price would you offer me for this?'

'Trade-in?[17]'

'No, cash.'

The man looked again at the car, made a sour face[18], and shook his head from side to side. 'Very hard to get rid of, these,' he said.

'It's a beautiful car,' Julian protested.

The man kept his sceptical face[19]. 'What is she, two-year-old?'

'Eighteen months.'

---

1. à côté de

2. pour traverser

3. La circulation était dense

4. une série de parkings de voitures d'occasion

5. sur des sites bombardés

6. dans les stations-service

7. empiétant sur les trottoirs

8. Il en choisit un assez grand

9. des modèles récents de voitures de qualité

10. pare-brise

11. son chiffon et son seau d'eau

12. Vous êtes bien matinal

13. patron

14. L'homme devint nettement plus froid

15. C'est moi

16. d'un geste de la main

17. C'est pour une reprise ?

18. prit un air revêche

19. sa mine sceptique

1. vendeur de voitures
2. carrosserie
3. Il passa le doigt sur une rayure
4. examina attentivement les pare-chocs
5. tâta les pneus
6. sur le marché
7. J'ai pas dit que je vous en donnerai des boutons de chemise
8. mon pote
9. la clé de contact
10. le moteur se mit en marche
11. Il renouvela l'opération
12. Elle a très peu de kilomètres au compteur
13. Mais est-ce qu'il est juste ?
14. Non.
15. s'insurgea Julian
16. Vous êtes dans quel domaine?
17. Chacun son métier, moi c'est les voitures et vous les foutus tableaux.
18. essayait de se contrôler
19. une lueur de triomphe

The car dealer[1] walked slowly around, examining the bodywork[2]. He fingered a scratch[3] in the door, looked closely at the bumpers[4], and felt the tyres[5].

'It's a beautiful car,' Julian repeated.

'That may be, but it don't mean I can sell it,' the man said. He opened the driver's door and got behind the wheel.

Julian felt exasperated. This was ridiculous. He knew very well the dealer could sell the Mercedes in the trade[6] if not on his own lot. It was just a question of how much the man would pay.

'I want cash,' he said.

'I haven't offered you shirt buttons for it[7] yet, mate[8],' the dealer replied. He turned the ignition key[9] and the engine fired[10]. He turned it off, let the engine die, and turned it on again. He repeated the process[11] several times.

'The mileage is very low[12],' Julian offered.

'But is it right?[13]'

'Of course.'

The man got out of the car and shut the door. 'I don't know,' he said.

'Do you want to drive it?'

'Nah.[14]'

'How the hell can you tell what it's worth without driving it?' Julian burst out[15].

The man remained cool. 'What business you in?[16]'

'I own an art gallery.'

'Right, then. I'll stick to motors and you stick to bleed'n' paintings.[17]'

Julian controlled his temper[18]. 'Well, are you going to make me an offer?'

'I suppose I could give you fifteen hundred for it, doing you a favour.'

'That's ridiculous! It must have cost five or six thousand new!' There was a flash of triumph[19] in the

118

dealer's eyes at that[1]. Julian realized he had given away[2] the fact that he did not know the original price of the car.

The dealer said: 'I suppose it is yours to sell[3]?'

'Of course.'

'Got the log-book?' Julian fished it out of his inside pocket and handed it over.

The dealer said: 'Funny name for a bloke[4], Sarah.'

'That's my wife.' Julian took out a card and handed it over. 'This is my name.'

The man put the card in a pocket. 'Pardon me asking, but she does know[5] you're selling it?'

Julian inwardly cursed[6] the man's canniness[7]. How could he guess? No doubt he figured[8] that for an art dealer to come to the East End to sell a nearly new Mercedes for cash there must be something faintly underhand going on[9].

He said: 'My wife died recently.'

'Fair enough.' The dealer obviously[10] did not believe the story. 'Well, I've told you what it's worth to me.'

'I couldn't let it go for much less than three thousand,' Julian said with a show of determination[11].

'I'll say sixteen hundred, and that's my top price[12].'

Julian decided he was expected to haggle[13]. 'Two-five,' he said.

The dealer turned his back[14] and began to walk away.

Julian panicked. 'All right,' he called out. 'Two thousand.'

'Sixteen-fifty, take it or leave it[15].'

'Cash?'

'What else?[16]'

Julian sighed. 'Very well.'

'Come into the office.'

1. à ces mots

2. qu'il venait de révéler

3. que vous êtes autorisé à la vendre

4. Drôle de nom pour un mec

5. elle est bien au courant

6. maudit en son for intérieur

7. perspicacité

8. Sans doute avait-il deviné

9. qu'il y avait peut-être anguille sous roche

10. de toute évidence

11. sur un ton qui se voulait déterminé

12. c'est ma meilleure offre

13. qu'il était censé marchander

14. tourna le dos

15. c'est à prendre ou à laisser

16. Bien sûr.

1. un bureau en bois déglingué
2. certificat de vente
3. vieux coffre-fort métallique
4. comptait la somme de 1 650 livres
5. en billets de cinq livres usagés
6. Alors qu'il s'apprêtait à partir
7. l'ignora
8. qu'il s'était fait avoir
9. Il chassa de son esprit cette rencontre désagréable
10. une euphorie maîtrisée
11. billets de cinq livres
12. Il se répéta
13. surgit derrière lui et le dépassa à toute allure
14. siffla et le héla
15. Il lui vint à l'esprit
16. elle découvrirait le pot aux roses
17. et remua les orteils
18. pour soulager la douleur
19. [ancien nom du siège de la police à Londres]
20. n'avait pas fait l'objet d'une déclaration de vol

Julian followed the man across the yard and into the old shop building which faced the main road. He sat at a battered wooden desk[1] and signed a sale certificate[2] while the dealer opened an old iron safe[3] and counted out £1,650[4] in used five-pound notes[5].

When he made to leave[6], the dealer offered a handshake. Julian snubbed him[7] and walked out. He was convinced he had been robbed[8].

He walked west, looking out for a taxi. He let the unpleasant encounter drift out of his mind[9], to be replaced by cautious elation[10]. At least he had the money – £1,650 in fivers[11]! It was plenty for his trip. He felt as if he had already started out.

He went over[12] the story he would tell Sarah. He could say he had been to see the decorators – no, it had better be someone she did not know. An artist who lived in Stepney. What was his name? John Smith would do – there must be plenty of real people called John Smith. He had gone into the house, and when he had come out an hour later the car had been stolen.

A cab came up behind him and flashed by[13], empty. Julian whistled and waved[14] but it did not stop. He resolved to be more alert.

It struck him that[15] Sarah might ring the police while he was away. Then the cat would be out of the bag[16]. He would have to give her the name of a nonexistent police station. A taxi came towards him, and he hailed it.

He stretched out his legs in the back of the cab, and wriggled his toes[17] inside his shoes to ease the soreness[18] from walking. All right, suppose Sarah rang Scotland Yard[19] when she discovered the station did not exist. They would tell her, eventually, that her car had not been reported stolen at all[20].

The whole scheme[1] appeared more and more fool-hardy[2] as he approached home. Sarah might accuse him of stealing her car. Could you be charged[3] with stealing from your wife? What about all that stuff in the marriage service[4] – all my worldly goods I thee endow[5], or something[6]. And there was a charge of wasting police time.

The taxi went along Victoria Embankment and through Westminster. The police would not bother to prosecute in a marital quarrel[7], Julian decided. But enough harm would be done if Sarah realized what he was up to[8]. As soon as she did, she would tell her father. Then Julian would be out of favour[9] with Lord Cardwell at the crucial moment when he might need money to buy the Modigliani.

He began to wish he had never thought of selling the car. What had seemed a brainwave[10] early that morning now looked like wrecking his chances of a find[11].

The taxi stopped outside the glass-walled house[12], and Julian paid the cabbie with one of the thick pile of fivers he had got from the garage man. As he walked up to the front door he tried desperately to think of a better yarn[13] to tell his wife. Nothing came[14].

He let himself quietly into the house. It was only just after eleven o'clock[15] – she would still be in bed. He made no noise as he entered the living room and sat down. He eased off[16] his shoes and sat back.

It might be better to go straight to Italy, now. He could leave a note saying he would be away for a few days. She would assume he had taken the car. When he came back he could spin her some tale[17].

Suddenly he frowned. Since he came in a small noise had been tugging at the sleeve of his mind[18], demanding attention[19]. He concentrated on it now,

1. Le plan tout entier
2. hasardeux
3. Pouvait-on être accusé
4. pendant la cérémonie du mariage
5. je te fais don de tous mes biens
6. ou quelque chose comme ça
7. d'engager des poursuites pour une querelle conjugale
8. ce qu'il mijotait
9. tomberait en disgrâce
10. un éclair de génie
11. semblait anéantir tout espoir de trouver une œuvre majeure
12. la maison aux baies vitrées
13. d'imaginer une histoire plus crédible
14. Mais il n'en trouva pas.
15. à peine onze heures passées
16. enleva délicatement
17. il lui raconterait un bobard quelconque
18. Depuis qu'il était entré dans la maison, un petit bruit l'interpellait
19. comme pour attirer son attention

and his frown deepened[1]. It was a kind of scuffling noise[2].

He sorted it into its components.[3] There was a rustle of sheets[4], a muffled creak of bedsprings[5], and a panting[6]. It was coming from the bedroom. He guessed Sarah was having a nightmare[7]. He was about to call out to wake her; then he remembered something about not waking people suddenly when they were dreaming. Or was that sleepwalking[8]? He decided to look at her.

He walked up the half-flight of stairs. The bedroom door was open. He looked in.

He stopped dead in his tracks[9], and his mouth fell open in surprise[10]. His heart beat very fast in shock[11], and he could hear a rushing noise[12] in his ears.

Sarah lay on her side on the sheets. Her neck was arched, her head flung back, and her expensively coiffed hair plastered[13] to her perspiring face. Her eyes were closed and her mouth was open, emitting low-pitched animal grunts[14].

A man lay beside her, his pelvis locked with hers[15] in a slow shudder[16]. The man's thick limbs[17] were dense with black hair. The muscles of his white buttocks bunched[18] and relaxed rhythmically. Sarah had one foot on the knee of the opposite leg, making a triangle; and the man squeezed the flesh of the inside of her raised thigh[19] as he murmured obscenities in a deep, clear voice.

On the bed behind Sarah lay a second man. He had blond hair, and his white face was slightly spotty. His hips and Sarah's bottom fitted together[20] like spoons in a drawer. One hand curled around Sarah's body and squeezed her breasts, one after the other.

It dawned on Julian[21] that the two men were making love to her at the same time. That accounted for[1] the curiously slow jerking[2] of the three bodies. He watched, appalled[3].

The blond man saw him and gave a giggle[4]. 'We've got an audience[5],' he said in a high voice.

The other man turned his head quickly, and they both stopped moving.

Sarah said: 'It's only my husband. Don't stop, you bastards, please.'

The dark man seized her hips[6] and began to jerk more powerfully than before. The three of them lost interest in Julian. Sarah said 'Oh yes,' again and again.

Julian turned away. He felt weak and sickened[7]; and something more. It was a long time[8] since he had seen that rutting look[9] on Sarah's face. He could not help but be aroused[10] by it. But the trace of sexual excitement was faint and uneasy[11].

He collapsed in the armchair again. They were making louder noises now, as if to mock him. His self-respect was demolished.

So that was what she needed to turn her on, he thought spitefully[12]. It wasn't my fault at all. Bitch, bitch. Julian's humiliation turned to vindictiveness[13].

He wanted to humiliate her, as she had him. He would tell the world about the cow and her sexual tastes[14], he would—

Christ.

Suddenly he was thinking very clearly. His head felt as if he had just taken a long draft of cold champagne. He sat still for a few seconds, thinking fast. There was so little time.

He opened the darkened glass[15] door of a cupboard against the wall and took out his Polaroid camera[16]. It was loaded.[17] He fitted[18] the flash attachment quickly, and checked that there were bulbs[19]. He set the focusing mechanism and the aperture[20].

1. *Cela expliquait*
2. *mouvement saccadé étrangement lent*
3. *horrifié*
4. *se mit à ricaner*
5. *Nous avons un spectateur*
6. *lui saisit les hanches*
7. *Un sentiment de malaise et d'écœurement s'empara de lui*
8. *Il y avait longtemps*
9. *expression lascive*
10. *Il ne put s'empêcher d'être excité*
11. *diffuse et assortie de gêne*
12. *C'était donc ça qu'il lui fallait pour être excitée, songea-t-il avec dédain*
13. *soif de vengeance*
14. *penchants sexuels*
15. *en verre fumé*
16. *appareil photo*
17. *Il était chargé.*
18. *fixa*
19. *ampoules*
20. *régla le zoom et l'ouverture du diaphragme*

1. sans se
montrer

2. devint de plus
en plus aigu et
de plus en plus
fort

3. se
transforma en
un hurlement

4. pénétra dans
la pièce

5. leva l'appareil
pour viser

6. viseur

7. déformés par
l'effort physique
ou l'extase

8. agrippant
avec frénésie
des poignées de
chair

9. actionna
l'obturateur

10. il y eut un
bref et vif éclat
de lumière

11. ne
semblèrent pas
le remarquer

12. tout en
réarmant la
pellicule

13. prit un
second cliché

14. chercha à
tâtons

15. carnet de
timbres

16. voleta

17. arracha la
pellicule exposée

18. clichés
instantanés

The voices from the bedroom turned into shouts as he jumped up the stairs. He waited outside the bedroom, out of sight[1], for a moment. Sarah made a noise deep in her throat which gradually rose in pitch and loudness[2]; a long, almost childlike cry. Julian knew that noise from the days when he had been able to make her do it.

As Sarah's cry turned into a scream[3] Julian stepped into the room[4] and raised the camera to his eye[5]. Through the viewfinder[6] he could see the three bodies moving in unison, their faces screwed up with exertion or ecstasy[7], their hands wildly grabbing fistfuls of flesh[8]. Julian pressed the shutter[9], and there was a momentary, bright flash[10]. The lovers did not seem to be aware of it[11].

He moved two steps closer, winding the film on as he went[12]. He lifted the camera again and took a second shot[13]. Then he moved sideways and took a third.

He went quickly out of the bedroom into the living room. He scrabbled[14] in a drawer and found an envelope. There was a book of stamps[15] beside it. He tore out twenty or thirty pence worth of stamps and stuck them on the envelope. He took a pen from his jacket pocket.

Where could he send it to? A piece of paper fluttered down[16] to the ground, having been dragged out of his pocket with the pen. He recognized it as the scrap on which he had written Samantha's address. He picked it up.

He wrote his own name on the envelope, then addressed it care of Samantha at the address on the scrap. He ripped the exposed film[17] in its paper wrapping out of the camera. He had bought the camera to photograph paintings. The film produced negatives as well as instant prints[18], but the negatives had to be immersed in water within eight minutes of the exposure[1]. Julian took the film to the kitchen and filled a plastic bowl[2] with water.

He drummed his fingers on the draining-board[3] in an agony of impatience[4] while the image took form on the celluloid.

Finally he returned to the living room, the wet[5] film in his hand. The dark man appeared at the bedroom door.

There was no time to put the pictures in the envelope. Julian dashed for the front door[6], and opened it just as the dark man caught up with him. He smashed the camera viciously into the man's face[7] and leaped out of the door[8].

He raced up the street.[9] The dark man was naked and could not follow. Julian stuffed[10] the negatives in the envelope, sealed it, and posted it in the post-box[11] on the pavement.

He looked at the prints. They were very clear.[12] All three faces could be seen, and there was no doubt about what they were doing.

Slowly, thoughtfully, Julian walked back to the house and let himself in. The voices from the bedroom were now raised in quarrelsome tones.[13] Julian slammed[14] the front door to make sure they knew he was there. He walked into the living room and sat down, looking at the photographs.

The dark man came out of the bedroom again, still naked. Sarah followed in a robe, and the spotty one came last[15], dressed only in a pair of obscenely small briefs[16].

The dark man wiped blood from his nose[17] with the back of his hand. He looked at the red smear on his knuckles[18], and said: 'I could kill you.'

1. dans les huit minutes suivant l'exposition

2. saladier

3. Il tapota des doigts sur l'égouttoir

4. dévoré d'impatience

5. humide

6. bondit vers la porte d'entrée

7. Il frappa violemment l'homme au visage avec l'appareil

8. et sortit de la maison en courant

9. Il remonta la rue à toutes jambes.

10. fourra

11. la cacheta et la posta dans la boîte aux lettres

12. Ils étaient très nets.

13. Dans la chambre, le ton montait, en querelle

14. claqua

15. le boutonneux ferma la marche

16. d'un slip si petit que c'était indécent

17. essuya son nez ensanglanté

18. la traînée rouge sur ses doigts

1. présenta
2. La haine enflamma les yeux brun foncé de l'homme.
3. Espèce de sale petit pervers
4. éclata de rire
5. son visage se figea dans un rictus sévère
6. Rhabille-toi, c'est chez moi ici !
7. serrant les poings et les relâchant
8. par intermittence
9. replia ses jambes sous son corps
10. briquet de table
11. corbeille à papier
12. en lieu sûr
13. une saharienne couleur fauve
14. pull à col roulé
15. s'adressa aux
16. et je ne veux pas le savoir
17. rien à craindre

18. [pantalon très large, en vogue à Oxford de 1920 à 1950]

Julian proffered[1] the photographs. 'You're very photogenic,' he mocked. Hatred blazed in the man's dark brown eyes.[2] He looked at the pictures.

'You filthy little pervert[3],' he said.

Julian burst out laughing[4].

The man said: 'What do you want?'

Julian stopped laughing, and set his face in a hard sneer[5]. He shouted: 'Get some fucking clothes on in my house![6]'

The man hesitated, his fists bunching and relaxing[7] spasmodically[8]. Then he turned on his heel and went back to the bedroom.

The other man sat on a chair and curled his legs up underneath him[9]. Sarah took a long cigarette from a box and lit it with a heavy table-lighter[10]. She picked up the photographs where the dark man had dropped them. She looked at them briefly, then tore them into small pieces and dropped them in a wastepaper basket[11].

Julian said: 'The negatives are in a safe place[12].'

There was a silence. The blond man seemed to be enjoying the excitement. Finally the dark man came back, dressed in a fawn safari jacket[13] and a white polo-necked sweater[14].

Julian addressed[15] the two men. 'I've nothing against you,' he said. 'I don't know who you are, and I don't want to[16]. You've nothing to fear[17] from these pictures. Never come into this house again, that's all. Now get out.'

The dark man went immediately. Julian waited while the other went into the bedroom, and came out a minute later, dressed in elegant Oxford bags[18] and a short blouson jacket.

When he had gone Sarah lit another cigarette. Eventually she said: 'I suppose you want money.'

Julian shook his head in negation[1]. 'I've taken it,' he said. Sarah looked at him in surprise.

'Before all . . . this?' she said.

'I sold your car,' he told her.

She showed no anger[2]. There was a faintly strange light[3] in her eyes which Julian could not interpret, and the trace of a smile at the corners of her mouth.

'You stole my car,' she said flatly.

'I suppose so. Technically, I'm not sure a man can steal from his wife[4].'

'And if I do something about it?'

'Such as?'

'I could ask my father.'

'And I could show him our happy family snapshots[5].'

She nodded, slowly, her face still unreadable[6]. 'I thought it would come down to that.[7]' She got up. 'I shall get dressed.[8]'

At the staircase she turned around and looked at him. 'Your note . . . You said you would be out all day. Did you plan all this? Did you know what you would find when you came back early[9]?'

'No,' he replied casually[10]. 'It was what you might call a lucky break[11].'

She nodded again, and went into the bedroom. After a moment Julian followed her.

'I'm going to Italy for a few days,' he told her.

'What for?' She slipped out of her robe[12], and sat in front of her mirror. She picked up a brush and began to run it through her hair[13].

'Business.' Julian looked at the large, proud globes of her breasts[14]. The image of her lying on the bed[15] with the two men came unbidden[16] into his mind: her neck arched, her eyes shut, her grunts of passion[17]. His eyes wandered[18] to her broad shoulders[19], her back narrowing sharply to her waist[20], the cleft at the base of her spine[21], the flesh of her buttocks

1. fit non de la tête
2. aucune colère
3. une petite lueur étrange
4. qu'un mari puisse voler sa femme
5. clichés
6. le visage toujours hermétique
7. Je pensais bien qu'il s'agirait de ça.
8. Je vais m'habiller.
9. en revenant plus tôt
10. avec désinvolture
11. un coup de chance
12. Elle laissa tomber son déshabillé
13. à se brosser les cheveux
14. ses seins ronds, imposants et fiers
15. Cette image d'elle, allongée sur le lit
16. surgit spontanément
17. ses gémissements de passion
18. Il promena son regard
19. ses épaules larges
20. qui s'affinait au niveau de la taille
21. le creux à la naissance de sa colonne vertébrale

flattened[1] on the stool. He felt his body stir in response to her nakedness[2].

He walked over and stood behind her[3], his hands on her shoulders, looking in the mirror at her breasts. The aureolae of her nipples[4] were dark and distended still, as they had been on the bed. He let his hands slide down[5] from her shoulders until they touched her breasts.

He pressed his body into her back, letting her feel the hardness of his penis[6], a vulgar signal that he wanted her[7]. She stood up and turned around.

He took her arm roughly[8] and led her over to sit on the bed. He pushed her shoulders.

Wordlessly, submissively[9], she lay back on the sheet and closed her eyes.

Chapter Four

Dunsford Lipsey was already awake[1] when the stout black telephone[2] beside his bed rang. He picked it up, listened to the night porter's hasty good morning[3], and put it down again. Then he got up and opened the window.

It looked out on to a yard[4], a few lock-up garages, and a brick wall. Lipsey turned away and looked around his hotel room. The carpet was slightly worn[5], the furniture a little shabby[6]; but the place was clean. The hotel was inexpensive[7]. Charles Lampeth, who was paying for the investigation, would not have quibbled[8] if Lipsey had stayed at the best hotel in Paris: but that was not Lipsey's style.

He took off his pyjama jacket, folded it on the pillow[9], and went to the bathroom. He thought about Charles Lampeth as he washed and shaved[10]. Like all the clients, he was under the impression[11] that a small army of detectives worked for the agency. In fact there were only half a dozen; and none of them could have done this job[12]. That was part of the reason[13] Lipsey was doing it himself.

But only part. The rest of the reason had something to do[14] with Lipsey's own interest in art[15]; and something to do with the smell of the case[16]. It was going to turn out to be interesting, he knew. There was an excitable girl, a lost masterpiece[17], and a secretive[18] art dealer- and there would be more, much more. Lipsey would enjoy untangling the whole thing[19]. The people in the case; their am-

1. réveillé

2. le gros téléphone noir

3. le bonjour lancé à la hâte par le portier de nuit

4. Elle donnait sur une cour

5. légèrement usée

6. un peu miteux

7. n'était pas cher

8. n'aurait pas ergoté

9. la plia sur l'oreiller

10. en faisant sa toilette et en se rasant

11. il était persuadé

12. aucun d'entre eux n'aurait pu faire ce travail

13. C'était la raison, entre autres, pour laquelle

14. Mais il le faisait aussi

15. en raison de son propre intérêt pour l'art

16. ce qu'il avait flairé dans ce dossier

17. un chef-d'œuvre perdu

18. discret

19. démêler l'affaire

bitions, their greed[1], their little personal betrayals[2] - Lipsey would know of them all before too long. He would do nothing with the knowledge[3], except find the picture; but he had long ago abandoned the straightforwardly utilitarian approach to investigation[4]. His way made it fun.[5]

He wiped his face, rinsed his razor, and packed it away in his shaving kit[6]. He rubbed a spot of Brylcreem[7] into his short black hair, and combed it back, with a neat parting[8].

He put on a plain[9] white shirt, a navy blue[10] tie, and a very old, beautifully made Savile Row suit - double-breasted, with wide lapels and a narrow waist[11]. He had had two pairs of trousers made with the jacket, so that the suit would last a lifetime[12]; and it showed every sign of meeting his expectations[13]. He knew very well that it was hopelessly out of fashion[14], and he was utterly indifferent to the fact.

At 7:45 he went downstairs to the dining room for breakfast. The solitary waiter brought him a wide cup of thick black coffee. He decided his diet would stand[15] bread for breakfast, but he drew the line at jam[16].

'*Vous avez du fromage, s'il vous plaît?*' he said.

'*Oui, monsieur.*' The waiter went away to get the cheese. Lipsey's French was slow, and badly accented; but it was clearly comprehensible.

He broke a roll[17] and buttered it sparingly[18]. As he ate, he allowed himself to plan the day. He had only three things: a postcard, an address, and a photograph of Dee Sleign. He took the photograph out of his wallet and laid it on the white tablecloth beside his plate.

It was an amateur picture[19], taken apparently at some kind of family gathering[20] – buffet tables on a lawn in the background[21] suggested a summer wedding. The style of the girl's dress indicated that it had been taken four or five years ago. She was laughing, and seemed to be tossing her hair back[1] over her right shoulder. Her teeth were not well shaped, and her open mouth was unbecoming[2]; but a personality of gaiety and – perhaps – intelligence came through[3]. The eyes had a turned-down look in the outer corners[4] – the reverse of Oriental slantedness[5].

Lipsey took out the postcard and laid it on top of the photograph. It showed a narrow street of high, shuttered[6] buildings. The ground floors of about half the houses had been turned into shops. It was an undistinguished street – presumably, postcard pictures of it could only be sold in the street itself. He turned it over. The girl's handwriting[7] told him much the same story[8] as her photograph had. In the top left-hand corner of the reverse side[9] of the postcard was the name of the street.

Finally, Lipsey took out his small orange-covered notebook. The sheets were blank[10] except for the first, which had written on it, in his own small handwriting, the address the girl was staying at[11] in Paris.

He would not confront her immediately, he decided. He finished his coffee and lit a small cigar. He would pursue the other line of enquiry[12] first.

He permitted himself an inaudible sigh. This was the tiresome part[13] of his work. He would have to knock on every door in the street of the postcard, and hope to come across[14] whatever had put Dee on the trail of the painting. He would have to try the side streets[15], too. His assessment of the girl led him to believe[16] she probably could not wait more than about five minutes before telling someone of her discovery.

Even if he was right, it was a long shot[17]. Her clue might have been something she saw[18] in a news-

1. rejeter ses cheveux en arrière
2. était peu esthétique
3. s'en dégageait
4. Les coins extérieurs de ses yeux retombaient
5. des yeux bridés
6. avec des volets
7. l'écriture
8. évoquait à peu près la même chose
9. du verso
10. vierges
11. où habitait la jeune fille
12. Il allait suivre l'autre piste
13. la partie fastidieuse
14. tomber sur
15. les rues adjacentes
16. Il pensait, selon son analyse de la jeune fille,
17. c'était hasardeux
18. Elle avait peut-être trouvé l'indice

paper; someone she met walking along the street; or something which happened to occur to her as she was passing through. The fact that her address was in a different part of Paris, and there seemed to be little in this area to attract her, was in Lipsey's favour[1]. Still[2], the probability was that he would spend a full day or more and get sore feet making a fruitless search.

He would make it all the same[3]. He was a thorough man.[4]

He gave another little sigh. Well, he would finish his cigar first.

Lipsey wrinkled his nostrils to exclude the smell[5] as he walked into the old-fashioned fish shop[6]. The cold black eyes of the fish gazed malevolently at him[7] from the slab[8], appearing alive[9] because, paradoxically, they seemed so dead in life.

The fishmonger[10] smiled at him. *'M'sieu?'*

Lipsey showed the photograph of Dee Sleign and enunciated[11], in his precise French: 'Have you seen this girl?'

The man narrowed his eyes, and his smile froze to a ritual grimace[12]. His face said that he smelled cops[13]. He wiped his hands on his apron[14] and took the picture, turning his back to Lipsey and holding it up to let the light hit it[15].

He turned back, handed over the photograph, and shrugged[16]. 'Sorry, I don't recognize her,' he said.

Lipsey thanked him and left the shop. He entered a narrow, dark doorway beside the fishmonger's[17] and climbed the stairs. The ache in the small of his back[18] intensified with the effort: he had been on his feet[19] for several hours. Soon he would stop for lunch, he thought. But he would drink no wine with

1. jouait en faveur de Lipsey
2. Néanmoins
3. quand même
4. Car il était minutieux.
5. serra les narines pour éviter l'odeur
6. la poissonnerie à l'ancienne
7. le fixaient d'un air malveillant
8. l'étal
9. et paraissaient vivants
10. poissonnier
11. formula sa question
12. se figea et fit place à une grimace de circonstance
13. qu'il avait reniflé la police
14. son tablier
15. tendant le bras pour l'exposer à la lumière
16. haussa les épaules
17. à côté de la poissonnerie
18. La douleur dans ses reins
19. il ne s'était pas assis

his meal – it would make the afternoon's trudging[1] insupportable.

The man who answered his knock on the door at the head of the stairs[2] was very old, and completely bald. He appeared with a smile on his face as if he would be glad to see the person who knocked, no matter who it was.

Lipsey caught a glimpse[3], over the man's shoulder, of a group of paintings on a wall. His heart jumped[4]: the paintings were valuable originals[5]. This could be his man.

He said: 'I am sorry to trouble you, m'sieu. Have you seen this girl?' He showed the photograph.

The old man took the photograph and went inside the flat, to look at it in the light, like the fishmonger. He said over his shoulder: 'Come in, if you will.'

Lipsey entered, and shut the door behind him. The room was very small, untidy, and smelly[6].

'Sit down, if you want,' the old man said. Lipsey did so[7], and the Frenchman sat opposite him[8]. He laid the photograph on the rough wooden table[9] between them. 'I am not sure,' he said. 'Why do you want to know?'

The wrinkled yellow face[10] was completely expressionless[11], but Lipsey was now sure that this man had put Dee on the track of the picture. 'Does the reason matter?[12]' he asked.

The old man laughed easily[13]. 'You are too old to be a wronged lover[14], I suppose,' he said. 'And you are very unlike her[15], so it is improbable that you are her father. I think you are a policeman.'

Lipsey recognized a mind as sharply analytical as his own[16]. 'Why, has she done something wrong[17]?'

'I have no idea. If she has, I am not going to put the police on her trail[18]. And if she has not, then there is no reason for you to pursue her[19].'

1. la marche
2. en haut de l'escalier
3. aperçut
4. Il eut un coup au cœur
5. des originaux de grande valeur
6. en désordre et sentait mauvais
7. s'exécuta
8. s'assit en face de lui
9. la table en bois rustique
10. Le visage jauni et ridé
11. dépourvu de toute expression
12. La raison importe-t-elle ?
13. rit de bon cœur
14. un amant trompé
15. vous ne lui ressemblez pas du tout
16. un esprit d'analyse aussi fin que le sien
17. quelque chose de mal
18. à ses trousses
19. vous n'avez aucune raison de la pourchasser

'I am a private detective,' Lipsey replied. 'The girl's mother has died, and the girl has disappeared. I have been hired by the family to find her and break the news to her[1].'

The black eyes twinkled. 'I suppose you might be telling the truth,' he said.

Lipsey made a mental note[2]. The man had given away the fact[3] that he was not in constant touch[4] with the girl: for if he had been[5], he would have known that she had not disappeared.

Unless she really had disappeared, Lipsey thought with a shock. Lord, the walking had tired him – he was not thinking clearly.

'When did you see her?'

'I have decided not to tell you.'

'This is very important.'

'I thought so.[6]'

Lipsey sighed. He would have to be a little rough[7]. In the few minutes he had been in the room, he had detected the smell of cannabis. 'Very well, old man. If you will not tell me, I shall have to inform the police that this room is being used for drug-taking[8].'

The man laughed with genuine amusement[9]. 'Do you think they do not know that already?' he said. His papery chuckle ran its course[10], and he coughed[11]. The twinkle had gone from his eyes when he spoke again. 'To be tricked into giving information to[12] a policeman, that would be foolish[13]. But to be black-mailed into it[14] would be dishonourable[15]. Please get out now.'

Lipsey saw that he had lost. He felt disappointed, and a little ashamed. He went out and closed the door on the old man's papery cough.

---

1. lui apprendre la nouvelle

2. prit note

3. avait laissé entendre

4. en contact permanent

5. car, s'il l'avait été

6. Je m'en doute bien.

7. un peu brutal

8. pour consommer de la drogue

9. sincèrement amusé

10. Son petit rire ténu s'égrena

11. il se mit à tousser

12. Se faire manipuler pour informer

13. idiot

14. le faire sous le chantage

15. déshonorant

At least there was no trudging to be done, Lipsey thought. He sat in a small restaurant, after a superb 12-franc lunch[1], smoking his second small cigar of the day. The steak, and the glass of red wine he had drunk with it, had made the world seem a little less depressing. Looking back[2], he realized that the morning had ruffled[3] him, and he wondered again if he were too old for fieldwork[4].

He ought to be philosophical[5] about such setbacks[6] now, he told himself. The break always came[7], if you waited long enough for it. Still, he had run into a dead end[8]. He now had only one line of enquiry[9], instead of two. His hand was forced.

He had to chase[10] the girl, rather than the picture.

He dropped his cigar in the ashtray, paid his bill[11], and left the restaurant.

A taxi pulled up[12] at the kerb outside, and a young man got out. Lipsey grabbed the cab[13] while the man was paying. He looked a second time at the young face, and realized he had seen it before.

He gave the driver the address at which Miss Sleign had been staying since June. As the car pulled away[14], he puzzled over the familiar face[15] of the young man. Putting names to faces was an obsession with Lipsey. If he could not match them, he felt a distinct professional unease[16], as if his ability was thrown into doubt[17].

He racked his brains[18] for a few moments, then came up with a name: Peter Usher. He was a successful young artist, and had some connection with Charles Lampeth. Ah yes, Lampeth's gallery showed his pictures. It was of no consequence[19]. Feeling easier[20], Lipsey dismissed[21] the young man from his mind.

The taxi dropped him[22] outside a small apartment block, about ten years old, and not very impressive.

1. un superbe déjeuner à 12 francs
2. En y repensant
3. désarçonné
4. travailler sur le terrain
5. Il devait prendre avec plus de philosophie
6. de tels contretemps
7. Le coup de chance finissait toujours par arriver
8. il se trouvait dans une impasse
9. piste d'investigation
10. se lancer à la poursuite
11. régla l'addition
12. s'arrêta
13. attrapa le taxi
14. s'éloignait
15. il réfléchit à ce visage familier
16. malaise
17. comme s'il doutait de ses compétences
18. Il se creusa la tête
19. sans importance
20. Rassuré
21. chassa
22. le déposa

Lipsey went in and bent his head to the concierge's window[1].

'Is there anyone at home[2] in number nine?' he asked with a smile.

'They are away,' the woman said, giving the information begrudgingly[3].

'Oh, good,' Lipsey said. 'I am an interior decorator[4] from England, and they asked me to give them an estimate[5] for the place. They said I was to ask you for[6] the key, and look over the place[7] while they were away. I was not sure if they would be gone yet.'

'I cannot give you the key. Besides, they have no right to redecorate without permission.'

'Of course!' Lipsey gave her his smile again, and turned on a certain middle-aged charm[8] which he knew he was capable of. 'Miss Sleign was most emphatic[9] that I should consult you, to get your advice and opinions.' As he spoke, he fumbled some notes out of his wallet[10] and into an envelope. 'She asked me to pass this to you[11], for your trouble[12].' He handed the envelope through the window, bending it slightly[13] in his hand to make the money crackle.

She took the bribe[14]. 'You must not take very long, because I will have to stay there with you all the time,' she said.

'Of course,' he smiled.

She hobbled out of her cubbyhole[15] and led him up the stairs, with a good deal of puffing and blowing[16], holding her back, and pausing for breath[17].

The apartment was not very large, and some of the furniture looked secondhand[18]. Lipsey looked around the living room. 'They were talking about emulsion paint[19] for the walls,' he said.

The concierge shuddered.

'Yes, I think you're right,' Lipsey said. 'A pleasant flowered wallpaper[20], perhaps, and a plain dark green carpet.' He paused in front of a ghastly side-board[1]. He rapped it[2] with his knuckles. 'Good quality,' he said. 'Not like this modern rubbish[3].' He took out a notebook and scribbled a few meaningless[4] lines in it.

'They didn't tell me where they were going,' he said conversationally. 'The South, I expect.'

'Italy.' The woman's face was still stern[5], but she enjoyed displaying her knowledge[6].

'Ah. Rome, I expect.'

The woman did not take that bait[7], and Lipsey assumed she did not know. He looked around the rest of the flat, his sharp eyes taking everything in[8] while he made inane remarks[9] to the concierge.

In the bedroom there was a telephone on a low bedside table. Lipsey looked closely at the scratch pad[10] beside it. A ballpoint pen lay across the blank sheet. The impression of the words which had been scribbled on the sheet above lay deep[11] in the pad. Lipsey put his body between the table and the concierge, and palmed the notebook[12].

He made a few more empty comments about the décor, then said: 'You have been most kind, madame. I will not keep you from your work any longer.'

She showed him[13] to the door of the block. Outside, he hurried to a stationer's[14] and bought a very soft pencil[15]. He sat at a sidewalk café[16], ordered coffee, and got out the stolen pad.

He rubbed the pencil gently over the impression in the paper[17]. When he had finished, the words were clear. It was the address of a hotel in Livorno, Italy.

*

Lipsey arrived at the hotel in the evening of the following day. It was a small, cheap place of about a

1. un horrible buffet bas

2. Il le tapota

3. ces meubles de pacotille modernes

4. incompréhensibles

5. maussade

6. divulguer ses informations

7. ne releva pas

8. ses yeux avisés remarquant chaque détail

9. qu'il débitait des inepties

10. bloc-notes

11. étaient gravés

12. cacha le bloc dans le creux de sa main

13. Elle le raccompagna

14. il se précipita dans une papeterie

15. un crayon à papier très gras

16. à la terrasse d'un café

17. les marques dans le papier

dozen bedrooms. It had once been the house of a large middle-class family, Lipsey guessed: now that the area was going down, it had been converted into a guesthouse[1] for commercial travellers[2].

He waited in the living room of the family's quarters while the wife went to fetch her husband from the upper regions[3] of the house. He was weary from travelling[4]: his head ached slightly, and he looked forward to dinner[5] and a soft bed. He thought about smoking a cigar, but refrained for the sake of politeness[6]. He glanced at the television from time to time. It was showing a very old English film which he had seen one evening in Chippenham. The sound was turned down.

The woman returned with the proprietor. He had a cigarette in the corner of his mouth. The handle of a hammer[7] stuck out[8] of one pocket, and there was a bag of nails[9] in his hand.

He looked annoyed at having been disturbed at his carpentry[10]. Lipsey gave him a fat bribe[11] and began to speak in stumbling, fractured Italian[12].

'I am trying to find a young lady who stayed here recently,' he said. He took out the picture of Dee Sleign, and gave it to the proprietor. 'This is the woman.[13] Do you remember her?'

The man looked briefly at the photograph and nodded assent[14]. 'She was alone,' he said, the inflection in his voice showing the disapproval of a good Catholic father for[15] young girls who stay in hotels alone[16].

'Alone?' said Lipsey, surprised. The concierge in Paris had given the impression the couple had gone away together. He went on: 'I am an English detective, hired[17] by her father to find her and persuade her to come home. She is younger than she looks,' he added by way of explanation[18].

---

1. pension de famille

2. représentants de commerce

3. quelque part dans les étages

4. Le voyage l'avait fatigué

5. il lui tardait de dîner

6. se ravisa par politesse

7. Le manche d'un marteau

8. dépassait

9. un sachet de clous

10. travaux de menuiserie

11. un gros bakchich

12. dans un italien hésitant et déstructuré

13. Il s'agit de cette femme.

14. hocha la tête affirmativement

15. qu'en bon père de famille catholique, il désapprouvait

16. qui séjournent seules dans des hôtels

17. engagé

18. ajouta–t–il, pour s'expliquer

The proprietor nodded. 'The man did not stay here,' he said with righteousness oozing from him[1]. 'He came along, paid her bill[2], and took her away[3].'

'Did she tell you what she was doing here?'

'She wanted to look at paintings. I told her that many of our art treasures were lost in the bombings.' He paused[4], and frowned in the effort to remember. 'She bought a tourist guide – she wanted to know where was the birthplace of Modigliani.'

'Ah!' It was a small gasp of satisfaction[5] from Lipsey.

'She booked a phone call to Paris when she was here. I think that is all I can tell you[6].'

'You don't know just where in the city she went[7]?'

'No.'

'How many days was she here?'

'Only one.'

'Did she say anything about where she was going next[8]?'

'Ah! Of course,' the man said. He paused to puff life into the dying cigarette[9] in his mouth; and grimaced at the taste of the smoke[10]. 'They came in and asked for a map[11].'

Lipsey leaned forward. Another lucky break[12], so soon, was almost too much to hope for[13]. 'Go on.'

'Let me see. They were going to take[14] the autostrada[15] to Firenze[16], then go across country to the Adriatic coast[17] – somewhere near Rimini. They mentioned[18] the name of a village – oh! Now I remember. It was Poglio.'

Lipsey took out his notebook. 'Spell it?[19]'

The proprietor obliged[20].

Lipsey got up. 'I am most grateful to you[21],' he said.

---

1. d'un air résolument rigide
2. a payé sa note
3. l'a emmenée
4. Il s'arrêta
5. un petit soupir de satisfaction
6. c'est tout ce que je peux vous dire
7. où elle est allée, exactement, en ville
8. où elle comptait se rendre ensuite
9. tira une bouffée pour raviver la cigarette
10. le goût de la fumée le fit grimacer
11. ont demandé une carte
12. Encore un coup de chance
13. c'était presque trop beau
14. Ils avaient l'intention de prendre
15. [autoroute, en italien]
16. [Florence, en italien]
17. de traverser le pays jusqu'à la côte adriatique
18. Ils ont cité
19. Vous pouvez épeler ?
20. s'exécuta
21. Je vous suis extrêmement reconnaissant

1. il s'arrêta sur le trottoir

2. pour respirer profondément

3. pour fêter ça

Outside, he stopped at the kerb[1] to breathe in[2] the warm evening air. So soon! he thought. He lit a small cigar to celebrate[3].

Chapter Five

The need to paint was like the smoker's craving for a cigarette[1]: Peter Usher was reminded of the time he had tried to give it up[2]. There was an elusive irritation[3], distinctly physical, but unattached to any specific part of his body. He knew, from past experience[4], that it was there because he had not worked for several days; and that the smell of a studio, the slight drag[5] on his fingers of oils being brushed across canvas[6], and the sight[7] of a new work taking place[8], were the only way of scratching it[9]. He felt bad because he had not painted for several days.

Besides, he was frightened.

The idea which had struck him and Mitch simultaneously, that drunken evening[10] in Clapham, had burst[11] with all the freshness and glory of a tropical dawn[12]. It had seemed simple, too: they would paint some fakes, sell them at astronomical prices, then tell the world what they had done.

It would be a gigantic raspberry blown[13] at the art world and its stuffed shirts[14]; a surefire publicity stunt[15]; a historical radical coup[16].

In the sobriety of the following days, working out[17] the details of the operation, they had realized that it would not be simple. Nevertheless it came to seem[18] more and more workable as they got down to the mechanics of the fraud[19].

But now, when he was about to take the first dishonest step on the way to the art swindle[20] of the century; when he was about to commit himself to

1. l'envie irrésistible d'une cigarette
2. pour Peter Usher, c'était comme à l'époque où il essayait d'arrêter de fumer
3. un vague sentiment d'irritation
4. par expérience
5. cette légère résistance
6. lorsqu'il appliquait la peinture à l'huile sur la toile
7. le spectacle
8. une nouvelle œuvre en formation
9. de s'en débarrasser
10. lors de cette soirée de beuverie
11. avait jailli
12. aurore
13. Cela serait un gigantesque pied de nez
14. et à tous ces prétentieux
15. un coup de pub imparable
16. un coup magistral et historique
17. en étudiant
18. elle s'était révélée
19. lorsqu'ils s'étaient attelés à la mécanique de l'escroquerie
20. la plus grande imposture artistique du siècle

a course[1] which would lead him well over[2] the line between protest and crime; when he was alone and nervous in Paris, he sat in an office at Meunier's and smoked cigarettes which did not give him comfort.

The graceful old building exacerbated his unease[3]. With its marbled pillars and high, stuccoed ceilings[4], it was too obviously a part of that confident, superior stratum of the art world – the society which embraced[5] Charles Lampeth and rejected Peter Usher. Meunier's were agents for half the top French artists[6] of the last 150 years. None of their clients were unknowns[7].

A small man in a well-worn[8] dark suit scurried purposefully across the hall[9] and through the open door of the room where Peter sat. He had the deliberately harassed look[10] of those who want the world to know just how overworked[11] they are.

'My name is Durand,' he said.

Peter stood up. 'Peter Usher. I am a painter from London, looking for a part-time job[12]. Can you help me?' He spoke only schoolboy French[13], but his accent was good.

A displeased look came over Durand's face. 'You will appreciate[14], Monsieur Usher, that we get many such requests from young art students in Paris.'

'I'm not a student. I graduated from the Slade—'

'Be that as it may[15],' Durand interrupted with an impatient motion of his hand. 'The company's policy is to help whenever we can.' It was plain[16] he did not approve of the policy. 'It depends entirely on whether we have a vacancy[17] at the time. Since almost all our staff require stringent security vetting[18], clearly there are few jobs for casual callers[19]. However, if you will come with me, I will find out whether we can use you[20].'

Peter followed Durand's brisk steps[1] across the hall to an old lift. The cage came creaking and grumbling down, and they got in and ascended three flights[2].

They went into a small office at the back of the building where a portly, pink-faced man[3] sat behind a desk. Durand spoke to the man in very rapid colloquial[4] French which Peter could not follow. The portly man appeared to have made a suggestion: Durand seemed to be turning it down. Eventually he turned to Peter.

'I am afraid I must disappoint you,' he said. 'We have a vacancy, but the job involves handling paintings[5], and we require references[6].'

'I can give you a telephone reference, if you don't mind calling London,' Peter blurted[7].

Durand smiled and shook his head. 'It would have to be someone we know, Monsieur Usher.'

'Charles Lampeth? He's a well-known dealer, and—'

'Of course, we know Monsieur Lampeth. Will he vouch for you?'[8] the portly man cut in[9].

'He will certainly confirm that I am a painter, and an honest man. His gallery handled my pictures for a while[10].'

The man behind the desk smiled. 'In that case, I am sure we can give you a job. If you would return tomorrow morning by which time[11] we will have called London—'

Durand said: 'The cost of the telephone call will have to be deducted from your wages[12].'

'That's all right,' Peter replied.

The portly man nodded in dismissal[13]. Durand said: 'I will show you out.' He did not bother to hide his disapproval.

Peter went straight to a bar and ordered a very expensive double whisky. Giving Lampeth's name had

1. emboîta le pas rapide de Durand

2. étages

3. un homme corpulent au visage couperosé

4. familier

5. implique la manutention de tableaux

6. nous exigeons des références

7. lâcha

8. Se porterait-il garant pour vous ?

9. l'interrompit

10. pendant quelques temps

11. entretemps

12. sera déduit de votre salaire

13. les congédia d'un signe de tête

143

been a foolish impulse[1]. Not that[2] the dealer would refuse to vouch for him: guilty conscience ought to see to that[3]. But it meant that Lampeth would know that Peter had been employed by Meunier's in Paris around this time—and that knowledge could do fatal damage to the plan[4]. It was unlikely; but it was an added risk.

Peter tossed off his whisky[5], cursed under his breath[6], and ordered another.

Peter started work the next day in the packing department[7]. He worked under an elderly, bent Parisian[8] who had devoted his life to taking care of pictures. They spent the morning uncrating newly arrived works[9], and the afternoon wrapping outgoing pictures[10] in layers of cotton wool, polystyrene, cardboard and straw[11]. Peter did the heavy work[12]: withdrawing nails from wood, and lifting heavy frames; while the old man prepared soft beds[13] for the pictures with as much care as if he were lining a cradle[14] for a newborn child.

They had a big, four-wheeled dolly[15] with pneumatic tyres on hydraulic suspension: the aluminium gleamed, and the old man was proud of it. It was used to transport the pictures around the building. The two of them would gingerly lift[16] a work on to its rack[17], then Peter would push it away, with the old man going ahead to open doors.

In a corner of the room where they did their packing was a small desk. Late on the first afternoon, while the old man was away at the lavatory[18], Peter went through all the drawers[19]. They contained very little: the blank forms[20] the old man filled up for each picture handled, a clutch[21] of ballpoint pens, a few forgotten paper clips[1], and some empty cigarette packets.

They worked very slowly, and the man talked to Peter about his life, and the pictures. He disliked most of the modern painting, he said, apart from a few primitives and – surprisingly, Peter thought – the super-realists[2]. His appreciation was untutored[3], but not naïve: Peter found it refreshing. He liked the man instantly, and the prospect of deceiving him became unwelcome[4].

On their trips around the building Peter saw plenty of the official company letterhead[5] on secretaries' desks. Unfortunately, the secretaries were always around, and so was the old man. In addition, the letterhead was not enough.

It was not until the end of the second day that Peter set eyes on the thing he had come to steal.

Late in the afternoon, a picture arrived by Jan Rep, an elderly Dutch painter living in Paris, for whom Meunier's were agents. Rep's work attracted huge sums[6], and he painted very slowly. A telephone call notified the old man that the painting was coming, and a few moments later he was instructed to take it immediately to the office of M. Alain Meunier, the senior of the three brothers[7] who ran the company.

When they lifted the picture out of the crate[8], the old man stared at it with a smile. 'Beautiful,' he said eventually[9]. 'Do you agree?'

'It doesn't appeal to me[10],' Peter said ruefully[11].

The old man nodded. 'Rep is an old man's painter[12], I think.'

They loaded it on to their dolly[13] and wheeled it[14] through the building, up in the lift, and into M. Meunier's office[15]. There they placed it on a steel easel[16] and stood back[17].

---

1. trombones

2. les surréalistes

3. Son jugement était celui d'un autodidacte

4. l'idée de le duper commençait à lui déplaire

5. papier à en-tête officiel de la société

6. pouvaient atteindre des sommes considérables

7. le plus âgé des trois frères

8. sortirent le tableau de sa caisse

9. dit-il, enfin

10. Il ne me plaît pas

11. avec regret

12. c'est un peintre qui plaît aux vieux

13. Ils le chargèrent sur le chariot

14. qu'ils poussèrent

15. jusque dans le bureau de M. Meunier

16. ils le placèrent sur un chevalet en acier

17. reculèrent

1. un homme à la mine grise et aux joues flasques
2. une lueur d'avidité
3. en se plaçant à une certaine distance
4. pour étudier le coup de pinceau
5. de chaque côté
6. grand bureau incrusté de cuir
7. en cristal
8. un porte-stylos de bureau
9. un petit tampon
10. Le regard de Peter se fixa
11. taché d'encre rouge
12. le manche était en bois poli
13. à l'envers
14. Ses doigts le démangeaient de s'en emparer
15. on remarquerait tout de suite sa disparition
16. à essayer de trouver un moyen
17. lui fut offerte sur un plateau
18. leva la tête
19. Tu sais où se trouvent les fournitures de bureau ?
20. Va me chercher des formulaires
21. je n'en ai presque plus

Alain Meunier was a grey, jowly man[1] in a dark suit, with – Peter thought – a glint of greed[2] in his small blue eyes. He looked at the new picture from a distance[3], and then walked close to study the brush-work[4]; then he viewed it from either side[5].

Peter stood near Meunier's huge leather-inlaid desk[6]. It bore three telephones, a cut-glass[7] ashtray, a cigar box, an executive penholder[8] made of red plastic (a present from the children?), a photograph of a woman – and a small rubber stamp[9].

Peter's eyes fastened[10] on the stamp. It was stained with red ink[11] at its rubber base, and the knob was of polished wood[12]. He tried to read the back-to-front[13] words of the stamp, but could only make out the name of the firm.

It was almost certain to be what he wanted.

His fingers itched to snatch it up[14] and stuff it into his pocket, but he was certain to be seen. Even if he did it while the backs of the others were turned, the stamp might be missed immediately[15] afterwards. There had to be a better way.

When Meunier spoke Peter gave a guilty start. 'You may leave this here,' the man said. His nod was dismissive.

Peter wheeled the dolly out through the door, and the two of them returned to their packing room.

He spent two more days trying to figure out a way[16] to get at the stamp on Meunier's desk. Then a better idea was handed to him on a plate[17].

The old man was sitting at his desk, filling out one of the forms, while Peter sipped a cup of coffee. The old man looked up from his work[18] to say: 'Do you know where the stationery supplies are?[19]'

Peter thought fast. 'Yes,' he lied.

The old man handed him a small key. 'Fetch me some more forms[20] – I have almost run out[21].'

Peter took the key and went. In the corridor he asked a passing messenger boy[1] where the supply room was. The boy directed him to the floor below[2].

He found it in an office which seemed to be a typing pool[3]. He had not been there before. One of the typists showed him a walk-in cupboard[4] in a corner. Peter opened the door, switched on the light, and went in.

He found a ream of the forms[5] he wanted straight away. His eye roamed the shelves[6] and lit on a stack of headed notepaper[7]. He broke a packet and took out thirty or forty sheets.

He could not see any rubber stamps.

There was a green steel cabinet[8] in the far end of the little room. Peter tried the door and found it locked. He opened a box of paper clips[9], took one, and bent it. Inserting it in the keyhole[10], he twisted it this way and that[11]. He began to perspire. In a moment the typists would wonder what was taking him so long.

With a click that sounded like a thunderclap[12] the door opened. The first thing Peter saw was an opened cardboard box[13] containing six rubber stamps. He turned one over and read the impression underneath.

He translated: 'Certified at Meunier[14], Paris.'

He suppressed his elation. How could he get the thing out of the building?

The stamp and the headed paper would make a suspiciously large package[15] to take past the security men[16] at the door on the way home. And he would have to conceal it from the old man[17] for the rest of the day.

He had a brainwave[18]. He took a penknife from his pocket[19] and slid its blade under the rubber bottom[20] of the stamp, working the knife[21] from side to

1. un garçon de courses
2. l'envoya à l'étage inférieur
3. un pool de dactylos
4. un cagibi
5. un paquet de formulaires
6. Il parcourut les étagères du regard
7. tomba sur une ramette de papier à en-tête
8. une armoire métallique verte
9. une boîte de trombones
10. serrure
11. il le fit tourner de tous les côtés
12. qui résonna comme un coup de tonnerre
13. boîte en carton
14. Certifié par Meunier
15. un paquet un peu trop grand
16. devant les hommes de la sécurité
17. faire en sorte que le vieil homme ne le voit pas
18. un éclair de génie
19. un canif dans sa poche
20. glissa la lame sous la base en caoutchouc
21. en maniant le couteau

side to dislodge[1] the rubber from the wood to which it was glued. His hands, slippery with sweat, could hardly grip[2] the polished wood.

'Can you find what you want?' a girl's voice came from behind his back.

He froze.[3] 'Thank you, I have them now,' he said. He did not look around. Footsteps retreated.[4]

The rubber came away from the bottom[5] of the stamp. Peter found a large envelope on a shelf. He put the notepaper and the thin slice of rubber[6] into the envelope and sealed it[7]. He took a pen from another box and wrote Mitch's name and address[8] on the envelope. Then he closed the steel cupboard door, picked up[9] his ream of forms, and went out.

At the last minute he remembered the bent paper clip[10]. He went back into the store, found it on the floor, and put it in his pocket.

He smiled at the typists as he left the office. Instead of going back to the old man, he wandered around the corridors[11] until he met another messenger boy.

'Could you tell me where I take this to be posted?' he asked. 'It's air mail.[12]'

'I'll take it for you,' the messenger said helpfully[13]. He looked at the envelope. 'It should have air mail written on it,' he said.

'Oh dear.'

'Don't worry – I'll see to it[14],' the boy said.

'Thank you.' Peter went back to the packing department.

The old man said: 'You took a long time.[15]'

'I lost my way[16],' Peter explained.

Three days later, in the evening at his cheap lodging house[17], Peter got a phone call[18] from London.

'It came,' said Mitch's voice.

'Thank Christ for that,' Peter replied. 'I'll be home tomorrow.'

Mad Mitch was sitting on the floor of the studio when Peter arrived, his fuzzy ginger hair[1] laid back against the wall. Three of Peter's canvases were stood in line on the opposite wall.[2] Mitch was studying them, with a frown on his brow[3] and a can of Long Life[4] in his hand.

Peter dumped his holdall on the floor[5] and went over to stand next to Mitch.

'You know, if anyone deserves to make a living out of paint, you do[6],' said Mitch.

'Thanks. Where's Anne?'

'Shopping.' Mitch heaved himself to his feet[7] and crossed to a paint-smeared table.[8] He picked up an envelope which Peter recognized. 'Clever idea, ripping[9] the rubber off the stamp,' he said. 'But why did you have to post it?'

'No other way to get the stuff out[10] of the building safely.'

'You mean the firm posted it[11]?'

Peter nodded.

'Jesus. I hope no one happened to notice[12] the name on the envelope. Did you leave any other give away clues?[13]'

'Yes.' Peter took the can from Mitch and drank a long draft of the beer. He wiped his mouth on his forearm[14] and handed the can back. 'I had to give Charles Lampeth's name as a reference.'

'Did they check it?'

'I think so. Anyway, they insisted on a referee they knew and could telephone.'

1. ses cheveux roux frisés

2. étaient alignées, debout contre le mur opposé

3. les sourcils froncés

4. une canette de bière Long Life

5. jeta son sac par terre

6. si quelqu'un mérite de vivre de sa peinture, c'est bien toi

7. se releva

8. table tachée de peinture

9. d'arracher

10. de sortir ça

11. que c'est l'entreprise qui l'a posté

12. que personne n'aura remarqué

13. As-tu laissé d'autres indices qui pourraient nous trahir ?

14. Il s'essuya la bouche sur son avant-bras

1. s'assit sur le bord de la table
2. que tu as laissé une piste grande comme l'autoroute M1
3. s'ils en avaient le temps
4. c'est qu'ils ne puissent pas nous trouver
5. Si tout se passe comme prévu.
6. Et de ton côté, comment ça s'est passé ?
7. Je me suis arrangé avec Arnaz
8. Qu'est-ce qu'il y gagne ?
9. Une bonne rigolade.
10. lança la canette et réussit à atteindre la corbeille
11. tombées du camion
12. Il a fait de l'argent à tour de bras
13. il a appris tout seul à apprécier l'art
14. se moque des pigeons
15. Un type relativement peu scrupuleux
16. il partage notre opinion du monde de l'art
17. Mille livres.
18. Qu'as-tu réussi à faire d'autre ?
19. sous de faux noms

Mitch sat on the edge of the table[1] and scratched his stomach. 'You realize you've left a trail like the bloody M1[2].'

'It's not that bad. It means they probably could trace us, given time[3]. Even then they couldn't prove anything. But what matters is they can't catch up with us[4] before we're finished. After all, we only want a few more days.'

'If everything goes to plan.[5]'

Peter turned away and sat on a low stool. 'How did your end go?[6]'

'Great.' Mitch brightened up suddenly. 'I swung it with Arnaz[7] – he's going to finance us.'

'What's in it for him?[8]' said Peter, curious.

'A laugh.[9] He's got a great sense of humour.'

'Tell me about him.'

Mitch swallowed the rest of the beer and threw the can accurately into a bin[10]. 'He's somewhere in his thirties, half-Irish and half-Mexican, brought up in the USA. Started selling original paintings out of the back of a truck[11] in the Midwest when he was about nineteen. Made money hand over fist[12], opened a gallery, taught himself to appreciate art[13]. Came over to Europe to buy, liked it and stayed.

'He's sold his galleries now. He's just a kind of intercontinental art entrepreneur – buys and sells, makes a pile, and laughs at the mugs[14] all the way to the bank. A moderately unscrupulous bloke[15], but he feels the same about the art scene as we do[16].'

'How much money has he put up?'

'A thousand quid.[17] But we can have more if we need it.'

Peter whistled. 'Nice guy. What else have you pulled off?[18]'

'I've opened us a bank account – under false names[19].'

'What names?'

'George Hollows and Philip Cox. They're colleagues of mine[1] at the college. For references, I gave the Principal and the College Secretary.'

'Isn't that dangerous?'

'No. There are over fifty lecturers[2] at the college, so the connection with me is pretty thin[3]. The bank would have written to the referees and asked whether Hollows and Cox were in fact lecturers[4] and lived at the addresses given. They will get told yes.'

'Suppose the referees mention it to Hollows or Cox?'

'They won't see them. It's four weeks to the new term[5], and I happen to know that they aren't social friends[6].'

Peter smiled. 'You have done well.' He heard the front door open, and Anne's voice called hello. 'Up here[7],' he shouted.

She came in and kissed him. 'I gather it went off all right[8],' she said. There was a sparkle of excitement[9] in her eyes.

'Well enough,' Peter replied. He looked back to Mitch. 'The next step is the grand tour[10], isn't it?'

'Yes. That's down to you[11], I think.'

Anne said: 'If you two don't need me, the baby does.' She went out.

'Why me?' said Peter.

'Anne and I mustn't be seen[12] in the galleries before delivery day[13].'

Peter nodded. 'Sure. Let's go over it[14], then.'

'I've listed the top ten galleries[15] here. You can get around them all in a day. You look first of all for what they've got plenty of[16] and what they're short of[17]. If we're going to offer them a picture[18], we might as well be sure[19] it's one they need.

---

1. Ce sont des collègues
2. plus de cinquante professeurs
3. il serait difficile d'établir un lien avec moi
4. étaient bien professeurs
5. On est encore à quatre semaines de la rentrée
6. en plus, je sais, qu'ils ne se voient pas
7. On est en haut
8. J'imagine que tout s'est bien passé
9. une lueur d'enthousiasme
10. La prochaine étape, c'est la grande tournée
11. Là, c'est à toi de jouer
12. ne devons pas nous montrer
13. avant le jour de la livraison
14. Voyons ça
15. les dix galeries les plus importantes
16. les œuvres qu'elles ont en grand nombre
17. ce qui leur manque
18. Quitte à leur proposer un tableau
19. autant être sûr

1. facile à
contrefaire

2. il faut qu'il
ait produit
beaucoup
d'œuvres

3. ses œuvres
ne doivent pas
toutes être
répertoriées

4. pour faire
sensation

5. que ça va
nous rapporter
au total

6. Une
atmosphère
studieuse

7. le gazouillis
de satisfaction

8. parc

9. En temps
normal, elle
aurait exigé
l'attention

10. parfois,
le couvercle
s'emboîtait

11. un stylo à
encre

12. une écriture
moulée

13. [livre d'art
de grand for-
mat, abondam-
ment illustré]

14. de
volumineux
ouvrages de
référence

'Secondly, the painter has to be easily forgeable[1]. He must be dead, he must have a large body of work[2], and there can be no complete record of his work[3] anywhere. We're not going to copy master-pieces – we're going to paint our own. You find one painter like that for each gallery, make a note, then go on to the next.'

'Yes – we'll also have to exclude anyone who ha-bitually used any specialized kinds of material. You know, everything would be much easier if we limit-ed ourselves to water-colours and drawing.'

'We couldn't raise the kind of money we need to make a spectacular splash[4].'

'How much d'you think we'll raise altogether[5]?'

'I shall be disappointed if it's less than half a million.'

An atmosphere of concentration[6] filled the big studio. Through the open windows, the warm Au-gust breeze brought distant traffic murmurs. For a long while the three people worked in a silence broken only by the contented gurgling[7] of the baby in a playpen[8] in the middle of the room.

The baby's name was Vibeke, and she was just a year old. Normally she would have demanded atten-tion[9] from the adults in the room; but today she was playing with a new toy, a plastic box. She found that sometimes the lid would go on[10], and sometimes it would not; and she was trying to figure out what made the difference. She too was concentrating.

Her mother sat nearby at a battered table, writ-ing with a fountain pen[11] in meticulous copperplate script[12] on a sheet of Meunier's letterhead. The table was littered with opened books: glamorous coffee table art books[13], heavy tomes of reference[14], and small learned articles in paper covers[1]. Occasionally Anne's tongue would stick out of the corner of her mouth as she laboured[2].

Mitch stood back from his canvas and gave a long sigh. He was working on a fairly large Cubist Picasso[3] of a bullfight[4]; one of the series of paintings which led up to the *Guernica*. There was a sketch on the floor beside his easel. He looked at it now, and deep frown-lines gouged his forehead[5]. He lifted his right hand and made a series of passes[6] at his canvas, painting a line in the air[7] until he thought he had it right; then with a quick final stroke he put the brush[8] to the canvas.

Anne heard the sigh, and looked up, first at Mitch and then at the canvas. A kind of stunned admiration[9] came over her face. 'Mitch, it's brilliant[10],' she said.

He smiled gratefully.

'Really, could *anyone* do that?' she added.

'No,' he said slowly. 'It's a specialized talent. Forgery[11] for artists is a bit like mimicry[12] for actors. Some of the greatest actors are lousy mimics[13]. It's just a trick which some people can do.'

Peter said: 'How are you getting on with those provenances?'

'I've done the Braque and the Munch, and I'm just finishing the Picasso,' Anne replied. 'What kind of pedigree[14] would your Van Gogh have?'

Peter was reworking the picture he had done in the Masterpiece Race. He had a book of colour plates open beside him, and he frequently flicked over a page. The colours on his canvas were dark, and the lines heavy[15]. The body of the gravedigger was powerful yet weary.

'It would have been painted[16] between 1880 and 1886,' Peter began. 'In his Dutch period.[17] Nobody

1. de petites brochures savantes
2. lorsqu'elle s'appliquait
3. un Picasso assez grand, de la période cubiste
4. une corrida
5. creusaient son front
6. réalisa une série de coups d'essai
7. en peignant une ligne imaginaire
8. d'un dernier coup de pinceau, il apporta la touche finale
9. Une sorte d'admiration mêlée de stupéfaction
10. impressionnant
11. La contrefaçon
12. l'imitation
13. de très mauvais imitateurs
14. provenance
15. le trait épais
16. Disons qu'il a été peint
17. Pendant sa période hollandaise.

1. je présume
2. un collectionneur fictif, à Bruxelles
3. Il apparaît aux mains d'un marchand
4. Pourquoi pas ?
5. Fais en sorte qu'il soit inconnu
6. un lavis gris pâle
7. la lumière fugitive norvégienne
8. omniprésente dans
9. de ressentir le froid
10. qu'il se mit à trembler
11. brisèrent le silence
12. se regardèrent, blêmes
13. stupéfaits et incrédules
14. le premier à se ressaisir
15. cache ces certificats d'origine
16. je retourne les toiles face contre le mur
17. le cœur au bord des lèvres
18. que les flics les aient déjà démasqués
19. agent de police
20. une moustache clairsemée

would have bought it then, I don't suppose[1]. Say it was in his possession – or better, his brother Theo's – for a few years. Then bought by some fictional collector in Brussels[2]. Turned up by a dealer[3] in the 1960s. You can invent the rest.'

'Shall I use the name of a real dealer?'

'Might as well[4] – only make him an obscure one[5]– German, say.'

'Mmm.' The room became quiet again as the three returned to their work. After a while Mitch took down his canvas and began a new one; a Munch. He put on a pale grey wash[6] over the whole surface, to get the brittle Norwegian light[7] which pervaded[8] so many of Munch's paintings. From time to time he closed his eyes and tried to rid his mind of the warm English sunshine in the studio. He tried to make himself feel cold[9], and succeeded so well that he shivered[10].

Three loud knocks at the front door shattered the silence[11].

Peter, Mitch and Anne looked at one another blankly[12]. Anne got up from the desk and went to the window. She turned to the men, her face white.

'It's a policeman,' she said.

They looked at her with astonished incredulity[13]. Mitch was the first to adjust[14].

'Go to the door, Peter,' he said. 'Anne, hide those provenances[15] and the notepaper and stamp. I'll turn the canvases with their faces to the walls[16]. Let's go!'

Peter walked slowly down the stairs, his heart in his mouth[17]. It just did not make sense – there was no way the law could be on to them already[18]. He opened the front door.

The policeman was a tall young constable[19] with short hair and a sparse moustache[20]. He said: 'Is that your car outside, sir?'

154

'Yes – I mean no,' Peter stuttered[1]. 'Which one?'

'The blue Mini with things painted all over the wings[2].'

'Ah – it belongs to a friend. He's a guest here[3] at the moment.'

'Perhaps you'd like[4] to tell him he's left his side-lights on[5],' said the bobby[6]. 'Good day, sir.' He turned away.

'Oh! Thank you!' Peter said.

He went back up the stairs. Anne and Mitch looked at him with fear in their eyes.

Peter said: 'He asked me to tell you that you've left your sidelights on, Mitch.'

There was a moment of uncomprehending silence.[7] Then all three of them burst out into a loud, almost hysterical laughter[8].

In her playpen, Vibeke looked up at the sudden noise. Her startled look dissolved into a smile[9], and she joined enthusiastically into the laughter[10], as if she perfectly understood the joke[11].

1. bégaya Peter

2. avec tous les trucs peints sur la carrosserie

3. C'est notre invité

4. Peut-être pourriez-vous

5. que ses feux de position sont restés allumés

6. [policier anglais, en uniforme et casque noirs]

7. Ils restèrent muets, ne comprenant pas.

8. rire hystérique

9. Son air étonné se transforma en sourire

10. elle se mit à rire aussi avec enthousiasme

11. avait parfaitement compris la plaisanterie

PART THREE

Figures in the Foreground

'You need to think of the role which pictures such as paintings have in our lives. This role is by no means a uniform one.'

LUDWIG WITTGENSTEIN,
philosopher

Chapter One

The multistorey, reinforced concrete hotel[1] in Rimini offered English breakfast[2]: bacon, eggs, and a pot of tea. Lipsey glimpsed a portion[3] on someone's table as he made his way through the dining room. The egg was fried hard[4] and there was a suspicious green patch[5] on the bacon. He sat down and ordered rolls and coffee.

He had arrived late last night and chosen his hotel badly[6]. This morning he was still tired. In the foyer he had bought the *Sun*[7] – the only English paper available[8]. He flicked through it while he waited for his breakfast. He sighed with exasperation: it was not his sort of newspaper.

The coffee made him feel a little less weary[9], although a real breakfast – the kind he cooked for himself[10] at home – would have been better. As he buttered his roll, he listened to the voices all around him, picking out accents[11] from Yorkshire, Liverpool, and London. There were one or two German voices, too; but no French or Italian. The Italians had more sense than to stay[12] in hotels they built for tourists; and no Frenchman in his right mind[13] would go to Italy for a holiday.

He finished his roll, drained his coffee[14], and postponed his cigar. He asked an English-speaking hotel porter for directions to the nearest car-hire office[15].

The Italians were feverishly turning[16] Rimini into a replica of Southend[17]. There were fish-and-chip restaurants[18], imitation pubs[19], hamburger bars

1. L'hôtel en béton armé, érigé sur plusieurs étages
2. proposait un petit déjeuner anglais
3. aperçut le contenu d'une assiette
4. trop cuit
5. une trace verte suspecte
6. avait mal choisi son hôtel
7. [tabloid anglais à très grand tirage]
8. le seul journal en anglais disponible
9. le revigora un peu
10. qu'il se préparait
11. en relevant les accents
12. n'étaient pas assez fous pour séjourner
13. aucun Français sain d'esprit
14. avala son café
15. l'agence de location de voitures la plus proche
16. s'employaient activement à transformer
17. [station balnéaire populaire au sud de Londres]
18. [vente à emporter de poisson/frites dans un cornet]
19. des imitations de pubs

and souvenir shops everywhere. Every spare plot of land[1] was a building site[2]. The streets were already crowded with holidaymakers[3]; the older ones in open-necked Bermuda shirts[4] with their wives in flowered dresses[5], and the younger, unmarried couples in bell-bottom jeans, smoking duty-free king-size Embassy.

He smoked his belated cigar[6] in the car-hire office, while a couple of officials[7] filled in lengthy forms and checked his passport and his international driving licence. The only car they had available at such short notice[8], they regretted, was a large Fiat in a metallic shade of light green[9]. The car was rather expensive, but as he drove it away Lipsey was thankful for its power and comfort.

He returned to his hotel and went up to his room. He studied himself in the mirror. In his sober English suit and heavy laced shoes[10], he looked too much like a policeman, he decided. He took his 35 millimetre camera in its leather case[11] from his luggage, and slung it around his neck by the strap[12]. Then he put a set of darkened shades[13] over the lenses[14] of his spectacles. He studied himself in the mirror again. Now he looked like a German tourist.

Before starting out, he consulted the maps which the hirers had thoughtfully provided in the glove compartment[15]. Poglio was about twenty miles away along the coast[16], and a couple of miles inland[17].

He drove out of the town and took a narrow, two-lane country road. He settled down to a leisurely 50 m.p.h[18], driving with the window open and enjoying the fresh air and the flattish, sparse countryside[19].

As he approached Poglio the road got even narrower[20], so that he had to stop and pull on to the shoulder[21] to allow a tractor to pass him. He stopped at a fork with no signpost[22], and hailed a farm worker in a faded cap and T-shirt, his trousers held up with string[1]. In halting[2] Italian, he asked for directions. The peasant's words were incomprehensible, but Lipsey memorized the gestures and followed them.

When he reached the village, there was nothing to indicate that this was Poglio. The small, white-washed houses were scattered about[3], some twenty yards from the road, some built right out to the kerb[4], as if they had been put up before there was any well-defined road there. At what Lipsey took to be the centre of the place, the road forked around a group of buildings leaning on one another for support[5]. A Coca-Cola sign outside one of the houses marked it as the village bar[6].

He drove through the village, and in no time at all found himself in the country again. He did a three-point turn[7] on the narrow road. On his way back he noticed another road off to the west[8]. Three roads into the village, for what it's worth, he thought.

He stopped again, beside an old woman carrying a basket. She was dressed all in black, and her lined face[9] was very white, as if she had spent her life keeping the sun off it[10].

'Is this Poglio?' said Lipsey.

She drew her hood back off her face[11] and looked at him suspiciously. 'Yes,' she said. She walked on.

Lipsey parked near the bar. It was just after ten o'clock, and the morning was beginning to get hot. On the steps outside the bar, an old man in a straw hat[12] was sitting, his walking stick across his knees[13], taking advantage of the shade[14].

Lipsey smiled and bid him good morning[15], then went past him up the steps[16] and into the bar. The place was dark, and smelled of pipe tobacco[17]. There

1. dont le pantalon était retenu par une ficelle

2. hésitant

3. étaient éparpillées

4. tout au bord de la route

5. qui s'adossaient les uns aux autres

6. indiquait que c'était le bistro du village

7. Il fit demi-tour

8. qui partait vers l'ouest

9. son visage ridé

10. à ne jamais l'exposer au soleil

11. Elle repoussa sa coiffe pour dégager son visage

12. avec un chapeau de paille

13. sa canne sur les genoux

14. profitant de l'ombre

15. le salua

16. les marches

17. sentait le tabac à pipe

were two tables, a few chairs, and a small bar with a stool in front of it. The little room was empty.

Lipsey sat on the stool and called: 'Anybody there?[1]' There were noises from the back of the place, where the family presumably lived[2]. He lit a cigar and waited.

Eventually[3] a young man in an open-necked shirt came through a curtain beside the bar[4]. He took in[5] Lipsey's clothes, his camera, and his shaded glasses with a quick, intelligent glance[6]. Then he smiled. 'Good morning, sir,' he said.

'I would like a cold beer, please.'

The barman opened a small household refrigerator[7] and took out a bottle. Condensation hazed the glass[8] as he poured.

Lipsey took out his wallet to pay. As he opened it, the photograph of Dee Sleign fell out on to the counter[9] and slipped over to the floor. The barman picked it up.

There was no glimmer of recognition on the man's face[10] as he looked at the picture, then handed it back to Lipsey. 'A beautiful girl,' he commented.

Lipsey smiled and handed over a note. The barman gave him change[11], then retired to the back of the house. Lipsey sipped his beer.

It looked as if Miss Sleign, with or without her boyfriend, had not yet arrived at Poglio. It was quite likely[12]: Lipsey had been hurrying, and they had not. They had no idea anyone else was after[13] the Modigliani.

Once again, he would have preferred to look for the picture rather than for the girl. But he did not know just[14] what had led her to Poglio. She might have been told that the picture was here; or that someone here knew where the picture was; or some more complex clue[15].

He finished his beer and decided to look around the village. When he left the bar the old man was still on the steps. There was no one else in sight.[1]

There was little enough to look at[2] in the place. The only other shop was a general store[3]; the only public building a tiny Renaissance church[4], built, Lipsey guessed, in some seventeenth-century flush of wealth[5]. There was no police station, no municipal office[6], no community hall[7]. Lipsey walked around slowly in the heat, amusing himself by drawing idle deductions[8] about the economics[9] of the village from its buildings and its layout[10].

An hour later he had exhausted the game's possibilities[11], and he still had not decided what to do. When he returned to the bar, he found that events had once again taken the decision out of his hands[12].

Outside the bar, parked near the steps where the old man still sat in the shade, was a bright blue Mercedes coupé with an open sun roof[13].

Lipsey stood looking at it, wondering what to do about it[14]. It was almost certainly Miss Sleign or her boyfriend, or both – nobody in the village would own such a car[15], and there was little reason for anyone else to come here. On the other hand, his impression was that neither she nor her boyfriend had a great deal of money – the Paris flat had indicated that much. Still, they might have been slumming[16].

The only way to find out was to go into the bar. Lipsey could not hang around outside looking casual[17]: in his suit and polished shoes he made an unconvincing village loafer[18]. He mounted the steps and pushed open the door.

The couple were sitting at one of the two tables, drinking what looked like long, iced apéritifs. They wore identical clothes: baggy, faded-blue trousers, and bright red vests[19]. The girl was attractive, but

1. Il n'y avait personne d'autre.
2. certes peu de chose à voir
3. un bazar
4. une toute petite église de style Renaissance
5. à quelque période faste du XVII s.
6. pas d'hôtel de ville
7. salle communale
8. en tirant de vaines conclusions
9. les finances
10. en observant ses bâtiments et sa disposition
11. il avait épuisé toutes les possibilités de son jeu
12. décidé à sa place
13. avec un toit ouvrant
14. Il l'observa en se demandant ce qu'il allait faire
15. ne possédait une telle voiture
16. ils étaient peut-être venus s'encanailler
17. traîner dehors, comme si de rien n'était
18. il pouvait difficilement passer pour le traîne-savates du village
19. des débardeurs rouge vif

the man was extremely handsome[1], Lipsey noted. He was a lot older[2] than Lipsey had expected – late thirties[3], perhaps.

They looked at Lipsey intently[4], as if they had been expecting him[5]. He gave them a casual nod and walked up to the bar.

'Another beer, sir?' the young barman asked.

'Please.'

The barman spoke to Miss Sleign. 'This is the gentleman I was telling you about[6],' he said.

Lipsey looked around, raising his eyebrows in an expression of amused curiosity[7].

The girl said: 'Have you got a picture of me in your wallet[8]?'

Lipsey laughed easily. He spoke in English: 'This man thinks all English girls look alike[9]. Actually, you do look a little like[10] my daughter. But it is only a superficial resemblance.'

The boyfriend said: 'May we see the picture?[11]' He had a deep voice with a North American accent.

'Surely.' Lipsey took out his wallet and searched[12] through it. 'Ah! It must be in the car.' He paid the barman for his beer, and said: 'Let me buy you two a drink.[13]'

'Thank you,' Miss Sleign said. 'Campari, for both of us.'

Lipsey waited for the barman to make the drinks and take them to the table. Then he said: 'It's odd[14], meeting another English tourist out here in the wilds[15]. Are you from London?'

'We live in Paris,' the girl said. She seemed to be the talkative one of the pair[16].

The boyfriend said: 'It is odd. What are you doing here?'

Lipsey smiled. 'I'm a bit of a loner[17],' he said with the air of one who makes something of a confession.

'When I'm on holiday, I like to get right off the beaten track[1]. I just get in the car and follow my nose[2] until I feel like stopping.'

'Where are you staying?'

'In Rimini. What about you – are you wanderers too[3]?'

The girl started to say something, but the man interrupted her. 'We're on a kind of treasure hunt[4],' he said.

Lipsey thanked his stars for the boyfriend's naïvety. 'How fascinating,' he said. 'What's at the end of it[5]?'

'A valuable painting, we hope.'

'Is it here, in Poglio?'

'Almost. There's a château five miles up the road.' He pointed south.[6] 'We think it's there. We're going there in a while.[7]'

Lipsey made his smile condescending.[8] 'Well, it makes a holiday exciting[9] – a bit out of the ordinary – even if you never find the treasure[10].'

'You bet.'

Lipsey drained his beer. 'Personally, I've seen enough of Poglio[11]. I'm moving on.'

'Let me buy you another beer.[12]'

'No, thanks. I'm in a car[13], and there's a long, thirsty day ahead[14].' He stood up. 'A pleasure to meet you. Goodbye.'

The Fiat was terribly hot inside, and Lipsey regretted not having the foresight to park it in the shade[15]. He wound his window down[16] and pulled away, letting the breeze cool him. He felt pleased: the couple had given him a lead[17], and let him get ahead of them. For the first time since he had started work on the case, he was on top of it[18].

He drove out on the southward road, in the direction the American had pointed. The road became

1. j'aime bien sortir des sentiers battus

2. je suis mon instinct

3. vous êtes aussi des aventuriers

4. une sorte de chasse au trésor

5. à l'arrivée

6. Il indiqua le sud.

7. Nous y allons dans un moment.

8. Lipsey sourit de manière condescendante.

9. cela rend les vacances plus palpitantes

10. même si vous ne trouvez jamais le trésor

11. j'en ai assez de Poglio

12. Permettez-moi de vous offrir une autre bière.

13. Je conduis

14. la journée va être longue et très chaude

15. de ne pas avoir pensé à se garer à l'ombre

16. Il baissa sa vitre

17. lui avait donné une piste

18. il avait une longueur d'avance

dusty[1]. He wound up[2] his window and turned on the car's air-conditioning at full blast[3]. When it was cool again, he stopped to look at his maps.

The large-scale chart[4] revealed that there was, indeed, a château to the south. It seemed more than five miles away – perhaps ten – but it was still quite conceivable that its postal address would be Poglio. It was slightly off the main road[5] – if main road it could be called – and Lipsey memorized the directions[6].

The journey took him half an hour, because of the poorness of the roads[7] and the absence of signposts. But when he arrived there was no mistaking the place[8]. It was a big house, built about the same time as the church in Poglio. It had three storeys, and there were fairy-tale towers[9] at the corners of the façade. Bits of the stonework were crumbling[10], and the windows were not clean. A separate stables building[11] had apparently been converted into a garage, and its doors stood open, revealing a petrol-driven lawn mower[12] and a very old Citroën station wagon.

Lipsey parked outside the gates and walked up the short drive[13]. Weeds grew in the gravel[14], and as he got closer to the house it looked more and more dilapidated[15].

As he stood looking up at the house, a door opened and an elderly woman walked towards him[16]. He wondered what approach to take.

'Good morning,' she said in Italian.

Her grey hair was neat, she was elegantly dressed[17], and the bones of her face indicated that she had once been beautiful[18]. Lipsey gave a small bow[19].

'I beg your pardon for this intrusion,' he said.

'Don't apologize.' She had switched to English. 'How can I help you?'

Lipsey had learned enough about her to decide on his approach. 'I wonder whether one is permitted to look around the outside[1] of this beautiful house.'

'Of course,' the woman smiled. 'It is pleasant to find someone interested[2]. I am the Contessa di Lanza.' She extended her hand, and Lipsey shook it, mentally revising his estimate of his chances of success[3] to around 90 per cent.

'Dunsford Lipsey, Contessa.'

She led him around to the side of the house. 'It was built in the first quarter of the seventeenth century[4], when all the land around here was given to the family as a reward for service[5] in some war or other. That was the time Renaissance architecture finally filtered through to the countryside[6].'

'Ah. Then it was built about the same time as the church[7] in Poglio.'

She nodded in agreement. 'Are you interested in architecture, Mr Lipsey?'

'I am interested in beauty[8], Contessa.'

He could see that she was suppressing a smile[9], and thinking that this stiffly formal Englishman[10] had a certain eccentric charm. That was what he wanted her to think.

She talked to him about the house as if she were retelling a familiar tale[11]; pointing out the place where the masons had run out of the right sort of stone and been forced to change, the new windows added in the eighteenth century, the small nineteenth-century west wing[12].

'Of course, we no longer own the district[13], and what land we have retained is rather poor[14]. As you can see, too many repairs have been postponed.' She turned to face him and gave him a self-deprecating smile[15]. 'Contessas are two a penny[16] in Italy, Mr Lipsey.'

1. s'il est possible de visiter l'extérieur

2. de voir que cela intéresse quelqu'un

3. ses chances de réussite

4. au début du XVIIe s.

5. en récompense de services rendus

6. est finalement parvenue dans les campagnes

7. environ à la même époque que l'église

8. Je m'intéresse à la beauté

9. qu'elle réprimait un sourire

10. que malgré son formalisme un peu guindé, cet Anglais

11. racontait toujours la même histoire

12. aile

13. nous ne possédons plus la région

14. est plutôt aride

15. un sourire peu indulgent envers elle-même

16. Des comtesses, il y en a beaucoup

'But not all have a family as old as yours.'

'No. The newer aristocrats are businessmen and industrialists. Their families have not had time to grow soft with living on inherited wealth[1].'

They had completed[2] the circuit of the house, and now stood in its shadow at the foot of one of the towers. Lipsey said: 'It is possible to grow soft on earned wealth, Contessa. I'm afraid I do not work very hard for my living[3].'

'May I ask what you do?'

'I have an antique shop[4] in London. It's in the Cromwell Road – you must visit next time you are in England. I'm rarely there myself.'

'Are you sure you wouldn't like to see the inside of the house?'

'Well, if it's not too much trouble[5] . . .'

'Not at all.' The Contessa led him through the front door. Lipsey felt the tingle at the back of his neck[6] which always came near the end of a case[7]. He had worked things just right[8]: he had gently given the Contessa the impression that he might be willing to buy something from her[9]. She was obviously in fairly desperate need of cash[10].

As she led him through the rooms of the house, his sharp eyes flitted quickly around the walls. There were a large number of paintings, mainly oil portraits of previous counts and water-colour[11] landscapes. The furniture was old, but not antique. Some of the rooms smelled unused[12], their aroma an odd mixture of mothballs and decay[13].

She led him up the staircase, and he realized that the landing was the showpiece of the place[14]. In its centre was a mildly erotic marble of a centaur and a girl in a sensual embrace[15]. The rugs on the highly polished floor were not worn. The walls all around were hung with paintings.

1. de se la couler douce en vivant de leur héritage

2. Ils avaient achevé

3. pour gagner ma vie

4. Je possède un magasin d'antiquités

5. si cela ne vous dérange pas trop

6. le frisson dans le cou

7. vers la fin d'une affaire

8. Il avait fait exactement ce qu'il fallait

9. qu'il voulait peut-être lui acheter quelque chose

10. Manifestement, elle avait besoin d'argent.

11. à l'aquarelle

12. sentaient le renfermé

13. un étrange mélange de naphtaline et de décomposition

14. la galerie du premier étage était le joyau de la maison

15. une étreinte sensuelle

'This is our modest art collection,' the Contessa was saying. 'It ought to have been sold long ago, but my late husband would not part with it[1]. And I have been postponing the day.'

That was as near an offer to sell[2] as the old lady would come, Lipsey thought. He dropped his pretence of casual interest[3] and began to examine the pictures.

He looked at each one from a distance, narrowing his eyes, searching for hints[4] of the Modigliani style: the elongated face, the characteristic nose which he could not help putting on women, the influence of African sculpture, the peculiar asymmetry. Then he moved closer and scrutinized[5] the signature. He looked at the frames of the pictures for signs of reframing[6]. He took a very powerful, pencil-beam torch[7] from his inside pocket and shone it on the paint, scanning for the giveaway traces[8] of overpainting[9].

Some of the paintings needed only a glance[10]; others required very close examination[11]. The Contessa watched patiently while he went around the four walls of the landing. Finally he turned to her.

'You have some fine pictures, Contessa,' he said.

She showed him quickly around the rest of the house[12], as if they both knew it was only a formality.

When they were back on the landing, she stopped. 'May I offer you some coffee?'

'Thank you.'

They went downstairs to a drawing room[13], and the Contessa excused herself to go to the kitchen and order coffee. Lipsey bit his lip as he waited[14]. There was no getting away from it[15]: none of the paintings was worth more than a few hundred pounds, and there were certainly no Modiglianis in the house.

1. mon défunt mari ne voulait pas s'en séparer
2. C'était la seule allusion à toute intention de vendre
3. Il cessa d'avoir l'air détaché
4. cherchant les indices
5. examina attentivement
6. pour voir si le tableau avait été réencadré
7. une petite lampe-torche très puissante
8. recherchant toutes traces qui trahivaient
9. une œuvre peinte par-dessus une autre
10. Pour certains tableaux, un seul coup d'œil suffisait
11. exigeaient un examen minutieux
12. Elle lui fit visiter rapidement le reste de la maison
13. salon
14. patienta en se mordant les lèvres
15. Inutile de se voiler la face

The Contessa returned. 'Smoke if you like[1],' she said.

'Thank you. I will.' Lipsey lit up a cigar. He took a card from his pocket: it bore only his name, business address, and telephone number – no indication of his trade[2]. 'May I give you my address?' he said. 'When you decide to sell your art collection, I have some acquaintances[3] in London who would like to know[4].'

Disappointment flashed briefly[5] on the Contessa's handsome face as she realized[6] that Lipsey was not going to buy anything.

'That is the full extent of your collection[7], I take it?' he said.

'Yes.'

'No pictures stored away in attics or basements?[8]'

'I'm afraid not.'

A servant came in with coffee on a tray, and the Contessa poured. She asked Lipsey questions about London, and the fashions, and the new shops and restaurants. He answered as best he could.

After exactly ten minutes of idle conversation[9], he emptied his coffee cup and stood up. 'You have been most kind[10], Contessa. Please get in touch next time you are in London.'

'I've enjoyed your company[11], Mr Lipsey.' She saw him to the front door.[12]

He walked quickly down the drive and got into the car. He reversed into the drive of the château, and caught a glimpse of the Contessa in his mirror[13], still standing in the doorway, before he pulled away.

He was most disappointed[14]. It seemed the whole thing had been in vain. If there had ever been a lost Modigliani at the château, it was not there now.

Of course, there was another possibility: one that, perhaps, he ought to have paid more attention to.

The American, Miss Sleign's boyfriend, might have deliberately sent him on a wild goose chase[1].

Could the man have suspected Lipsey? Well, it was a possibility; and Lipsey believed that possibilities were there to be exhausted[2]. He sighed as he made his decision: he would have to keep track of the couple[3] until he was sure that they, too, had given up.

He was not quite sure how to set about trailing them now[4]. He could hardly follow them around[5], as he might have in a city. He would have to ask after them[6].

He returned to Poglio by a slightly different route[7], heading for the third road from the village[8]: the one which entered from the west. About a mile outside Poglio he spotted a house[9] near the road with a beer advertisement in the window. Outside was one small circular iron table. It looked like a bar.

Lipsey was hungry and thirsty[10]. He pulled off the road on to the baked-earth parking lot[11] in front of the place and killed the engine[12].

1. mis sur une fausse piste
2. que toute possibilité devait être envisagée
3. filer le couple
4. comment organiser leur filature, à présent
5. Il ne pouvait pas les suivre partout
6. s'informer de leurs moindres faits et gestes
7. en changeant légèrement d'itinéraire
8. en direction de la troisième route partant du village
9. il remarqua une maison
10. avait faim et soif
11. s'engagea sur la terre craquelée du parking
12. coupa le moteur

Chapter Two

'You fat liar[1], Mike!' exclaimed Dee. Her eyes were wide with pretended horror.[2]

His full lips[3] curled in a grin, but his eyes did not smile. 'You can't afford scruples[4] when you're dealing with that type[5].'

'What type? I thought he was a rather nice fellow[6]. Bit dull[7], I suppose.'

Mike sipped at his fifth Campari, and lit a fresh cigarette. He smoked long Pall Mall without filters, and Dee suspected that was how he got his emery-board voice[8]. He blew out smoke and said: 'Just being here at the same time as us[9] was a big coincidence. I mean, nobody would come here[10], not even a wandering loner[11]. But the picture clinched it[12]. All that stuff about his daughter was a bit of quick improvisation. He was looking for you.'

'I was afraid you'd say that.' Dee took his cigarette and sucked on it, then handed it back.

'You're sure you've never seen him before?'

'Sure.'

'All right. Now think[13]: who might have known[14] about the Modigliani?'

'Do you think that's it? Somebody else is after the picture? It's a bit melodramatic.'

'The hell it is.[15] Listen, darling, in the art world, word of this sort of thing spreads[16] like VD[17] in Times Square. Now who have you told?'

'Well, Claire, I suppose. At least, I may have mentioned it to her while she was in the flat.'

172

'She doesn't really count. Did you write home?[1]'

'Oh, God, yes. I wrote to Sammy.'

'Who's he?'

'The actress – Samantha Winacre.'

'I've heard of her. I didn't know you knew her.'

'I don't see her a lot[2], but we get on well when I do. We were at school together. She's older than me, but she got her schooling late[3]. I think her father went around the world, or something.'

'Is she an art buff?[4]'

'Not as far as I know. But I expect she's got arty friends[5].'

'Anybody else?'

'Yes.' Dee hesitated.

'Shoot.[6]'

'Uncle Charlie.'

'The dealer?'

Dee nodded wordlessly.

'Jeeze[7],' Mike sighed. 'That ties it up in a ribbon.[8]'

Dee was shocked. 'You think Uncle Charles would really try to find my picture before I do[9]?'

'He's a dealer[10], isn't he? He'd do anything, including trade his mom[11], for a find.'

'The old sod.[12] Anyway, you've sent that undertaker[13] on a wild goose chase.'

'It ought to keep him busy for a while.[14]'

Dee grinned. 'Is there a château five miles south of here?'

'Hell, I don't know.[15] He's sure to find one sooner or later.[16] Then he'll waste a lot of time[17] trying to get in, and looking for Modiglianis.' Mike stood up. 'Which gives us a chance to get a start on him[18].'

He paid the bill and they walked out into the glaring sunshine[19]. Dee said: 'I think the church is the best place to start. Vicars[20] always seem to know everything about everybody.'

1. As-tu écrit en Angleterre ?

2. Je ne la vois pas beaucoup

3. elle a commencé à aller à l'école un peu tard

4. C'est une mordue de l'art ?

5. certains de ses amis sont des artistes

6. Dis-moi

7. Bon sang !

8. Tout s'explique.

9. avant moi

10. C'est un marchand d'art

11. Il ferait n'importe quoi, même vendre sa propre mère

12. Le vieil enfoiré.

13. croque-mort

14. Ça devrait l'occuper pendant un moment.

15. Ça, je n'en ai pas la moindre idée.

16. Il en trouvera bien un tôt ou tard.

17. il va perdre beaucoup de temps

18. d'avoir un coup d'avance sur lui

19. soleil éblouissant

20. Les pasteurs

'Priests, in Italy[1],' Mike corrected her. He had been brought up a Catholic[2].

They walked hand in hand along the main street. The oppressive heat seemed to impose on them[3] the enervated lifestyle[4] of the village: they moved slowly and spoke little[5], subconsciously adjusting to the climate[6].

They arrived at the pretty little church, and stood in its shade for a few minutes, enjoying the cool. Mike said: 'Have you thought about what you're going to do with the picture if you get it?'

'Yes, I've thought a lot,' she replied. She wrinkled the bridge of her nose[7] in a frown which was all her own[8]. 'Most of all[9], I want to study it. It ought to provide enough ideas for half a thesis[10] – and the rest is just padding[11]. But . . .'

'But what?'

'You tell me but what.'

'The money.'

'Damn right.[12] Oops!' She caught herself swearing, and looked around the churchyard nervously.

'There's a lot of it involved.[13]'

'Money? I know.' She tossed her hair back over her shoulder. 'I'm not trying to kid myself I'm not interested in cash, either. Perhaps if we could sell it[14] to someone who would let me see it whenever I wanted – maybe a museum.'

Mike said levelly[15]: 'I notice you said "we".'

'Of course! You're in this with me, aren't you?[16]'

He put his hands on her shoulders. 'You only just invited me.[17]' He kissed her lips quickly. 'You have just hired an agent.[18] I think you made a very good choice.'

She laughed. 'What do you think I ought to do about marketing it[19]?'

'I'm not sure. I've got some ideas kicking around in my mind[1], but nothing definite. Let's find the painting first.'

They entered the church and looked around. Dee stepped out of her sandals and squirmed her hot feet[2] on the cold stone floors. At the other end of the nave, a robed priest[3] was performing a solitary ceremony. Dee and Mike waited silently for him to finish.

Eventually he approached them[4], a welcoming smile on his broad peasant's face.

Dee murmured: 'I wonder if you can help us, Father.'

When he got close, they realized he was not as young as his boyishly short haircut[5] made him seem from a distance. 'I hope so,' he said. He spoke at normal volume, but his voice boomed in the still emptiness of the church[6]. 'I suspect it is secular help you want[7], much as I might wish it otherwise. Am I right?[8]'

Dee nodded.

'Then let us step outside[9].' He took their elbows[10], one in each hand, and pushed them gently through the door. Outside, he glanced up into the sky. 'Thank God for wonderful sunshine[11],' he said. 'Although you should be careful, my dear, with your complexion. What can I do for you?'

'We're trying to trace a man,' Dee began. 'His name was Danielli. He was a rabbi, from Livorno, and we think he moved to Poglio[12] in about 1920. He was ill, and not young, so he probably died soon after.'

The priest frowned and shook his head. 'I have never heard the name. It was certainly before my time – I wasn't born in 1920. And if he was Jewish, I don't suppose the Church buried him[13], so we will have no records[14].'

1. quelques idées qui me trottent dans la tête

2. tortilla ses pieds brûlants

3. un prêtre en tenue

4. il vint à leur rencontre

5. sa coupe de cheveux enfantine

6. résonnait dans l'église déserte et silencieuse

7. que c'est une aide laïque qu'il vous faut

8. N'est-ce pas ?

9. allons à l'extérieur

10. Les tenant par le coude

11. Merci Seigneur pour ce soleil radieux

12. qu'il s'est installé à Poglio

13. je ne pense pas qu'il ait eu un enterrement catholique

14. nous n'en aurons aucune trace

'You have never even heard him talked about[1]?'

'No. And there is certainly no Danielli family in Poglio. However, others in the village have longer memories than mine[2]. And no one can hide in such a small place.' He looked at them hesitantly for a moment, as if making up his mind about something. 'Who told you he came here?'

'Another rabbi – in Livorno.' Dee realized the priest was desperately curious to know[3] why they were interested in the man.

He hesitated again, then asked: 'Are you related to him?[4]'

'No.' Dee looked at Mike, who gave a quick nod. 'We're actually trying to trace a picture which we think he had.'

'Ah.' The priest was satisfied. 'Well, Poglio is an unlikely place to find a masterpiece; but I wish you well[5].' He shook their hands, then turned back into his church.

The couple walked back towards the village[6]. 'A nice man[7],' Dee said lazily[8].

'And a nice church. Dee, shall we get married in a church[9]?'

She stopped and turned to look at him. 'Married?[10]'

'Don't you want to marry me?'

'You only just invited me[11] – but I think you made a very good choice.'

He laughed, and shrugged his shoulders in embarrassment[12]. 'It just kind of slipped out[13],' he said.

Dee kissed him affectionately. 'There was a certain boyish charm about it[14],' she said.

'Well, since I seem to have asked you . . .'

'Mike, if it's anyone, it's you[15]. But I don't know whether I want to marry anyone at all[16].'

'There's a certain girlish charm about that,' he said. 'One all.[17]'

176

She took his hand and they walked on. 'Why don't you ask for something a bit less ambitious[1]?'

'Such as?'

'Ask me to live with you for a couple of years to see how it works out[2].'

'So you can have your evil way with me[3], then leave me without any visible means of support[4]?'

'Yes.'

This time he stopped her. 'Dee, we always turn everything into a joke. It's our way of keeping our relationship in an emotionally low key[5]. That's why we suddenly start talking about our future together at a crazy time like this[6]. But I love you, and I want you to live with me.'

'It's all because of my picture[7], isn't it.' She smiled.

'C'mon.[8]'

Her face became very serious. She said quietly: 'Yes, Mike, I'd like to live with you.'

He wound his long arms around her and kissed her mouth, slowly this time. A village woman walked by and averted her face from the scandal[9]. Eventually Dee whispered: 'We could get arrested for this.'

They walked even more slowly, his arm around her shoulders and hers about his waist. Dee said: 'Where shall we live?'

Mike looked startled. 'What's wrong with South Street?'

'It's a scruffy bachelor pad, that's what.[10]'

'Nuts. It's big, it's right in the centre of Mayfair.'

She smiled. 'I knew you hadn't thought much about it. Mike, I want to set up home with you[11], not just move into your place[12].'

'Mmm.' He looked thoughtful.[13]

'The apartment is knee-deep in rubbish[14], it needs decorating, and the kitchen is pokey[15]. The furniture is all odds and sods[16]—'

1. quelque chose de moins ambitieux

2. pour voir comment ça se passe

3. que tu fasses de moi tout ce que tu veux

4. sans aucun moyen de subsistance

5. de ne pas nous laisser emballer par la passion

6. à un moment aussi insensé

7. Tout ça à cause de mon tableau

8. Mais non.

9. détourna le regard de ce spectacle scandaleux

10. Ce n'est qu'une garçonnière miteuse, voilà.

11. m'installer avec toi

12. emménager chez toi

13. Il prit un air pensif.

14. rempli d'ordures

15. la cuisine est exiguë

16. un bric-à-brac

'So what would you like? A three-bedroomed semi[1] in Fulham? A town house[2] in Ealing? A mansion[3] in Surrey?'

'Somewhere light and spacious, with a view of a park[4], but near the centre.'

'I have a feeling you've got somewhere in mind.'

'Regent's Park.'

Mike laughed. 'Hell, how long have you been planning this?'

'Didn't you know I was a gold-digger[5]?' She smiled up into his eyes, and he bent his head to kiss her again.

'You shall have it,' he said. 'A new place[6] – you can get it decorated and furnished[7] when we get back to town—'

'Slow down! We don't know if there'll be a flat vacant there[8].'

'We'll get one.'

They stopped beside the car, and leaned against the hot paintwork[9]. Dee turned her face up to the sun. 'How long ago did you decide . . . about this?'

'I don't think I decided at all. It just gradually grew in my mind – the idea of spending my life with you. By the time I noticed, I was already too far gone to alter it[10].'

'Funny.[11]'

'Why?'

'It was just the reverse[12] with me.'

'When did you decide?'

'When I saw your car outside the hotel at Livorno. Funny that you should ask me so soon afterwards[13].' She opened her eyes and lowered her head. 'I'm glad you did.'

They looked at each other silently for a minute. Mike said: 'This is crazy. We're supposed to be hot on the trail[1] of an art find[2], and here we are looking cow-eyed at each other[3].'

Dee giggled. 'All right. Let's ask the old man.'

The man with the straw hat and the walking-stick moved with the shade[4], from the steps of the bar to a doorway around the corner. But he looked so completely still[5] that Dee found herself imagining that he had been levitated[6] from the one place to the other without actually moving a muscle. As they got close to him[7], they realized that his eyes belied his lifelessness[8]: they were small and darting[9], and a peculiar shade of green[10].

Dee said: 'Good morning, sir. Can you tell me whether there is a family named Danielli in Poglio?'

The old man shook his head. Dee was not sure if he meant there was no such family, or simply that he did not know. Mike touched her elbow, then walked quickly around the corner in the direction of the bar.

Dee crouched beside the old man[11] in the doorway and flashed a smile[12]. 'You must have a long memory[13],' she said.

He mellowed slightly[14], and nodded his head.

'Were you here in 1920?'

He gave a short laugh. 'Before then – well before[15].'

Mike came hurrying back[16] with a glass in his hand. 'The barman says he drinks absinthe,' he explained in English. He handed the glass to the old man, who took it and drained it in one swallow[17].

Dee also spoke in English. 'It's a pretty crude form of persuasion[18],' she said distastefully[19].

'Nuts. The barman says he's been waiting here all morning for some of the tourists to buy him a drink. That's the only reason he's sitting there.'

Dee switched to Italian. 'Do you remember back to about 1920?[20]'

---

1. à la poursuite
2. d'un chef-d'œuvre disparu
3. à nous faire les yeux doux
4. se déplaçait en fonction de l'ombre
5. si parfaitement immobile
6. qu'il avait été soulevé par lévitation
7. En se rapprochant de lui
8. ses yeux contredisaient sa torpeur
9. petits et perçants
10. d'un vert particulier
11. s'accroupit à côté du vieil homme
12. lui adressa un sourire
13. une mémoire qui remonte loin
14. se radoucit
15. bien avant ça
16. revint à toute allure
17. l'avala cul-sec
18. C'est plutôt raide comme moyen de persuasion
19. d'un air contrarié
20. Vos souvenirs remontent-ils jusqu'à environ 1920 ?

1. des étrangers qui se seraient installés dans le village
2. Ils étaient nombreux.
3. exaspéré
4. Il arrivait au bout de son maigre vocabulaire italien.
5. sur la route qui va vers l'ouest, en sortant du village
6. Putain, pourquoi
7. espèce de petit con
8. Il ricanait joyeusement
9. Il se releva péniblement
10. partit en boitillant
11. pour frapper le trottoir avec sa canne
12. C'était contagieux
13. Je suis un vrai pigeon
14. qu'on ferait bien de trouver ce bar
15. Si tu insistes.
16. son visage se fendit d'un grand sourire
17. pour vous jouer ce tour
18. qu'une fois par an, à peu près

'Yes,' the old man said slowly.

'Was there a Danielli family here then?' Mike asked impatiently.

'No.'

'Do you remember any strangers moving to the village[1] around that time?'

'Quite a few.[2] There was a war, you know.'

Mike looked at Dee in exasperation[3]. He said: 'Are there any Jewish people in the village?' His skimpy Italian was running out.[4]

'Yes. They keep the bar on the west road out of the village[5]. That's where Danielli lived when he was alive.'

They looked at the old man in astonishment. Mike turned to Dee and said in English: 'Why in hell[6] didn't he tell us that at the start?'

'Because you didn't ask me, you young cunt[7],' the man said in English. He cackled merrily[8], pleased with his joke. He struggled to his feet[9] and hobbled off[10] down the road, still cackling; stopping now and then to bang his stick on the pavement[11] and laugh even louder.

Mike's face was comical, and Dee too burst out laughing. It was infectious[12], and Mike laughed at himself. 'Talk about a sucker[13],' he said.

'I suppose we'd better find the bar[14] on the west road out of town,' Dee suggested.

'It's hot. Let's have a drink first.'

'Twist my arm.[15]'

They walked into the cool of the bar again. The young barman was waiting behind the bar. When he saw them his face split in a wide grin[16].

'You knew!' Dee accused him.

'I confess it,' he said. 'He wasn't really waiting to be bought drinks. He was waiting to play that trick[17]. We have tourists here only about once a year[18], and

it's the high spot of the year[1] for him. Tonight he
will be in here, telling the story to anyone who'll
listen[2].'

'Two Camparis, please,' Mike said.

1. l'évènement de
l'année

2. à qui voudra
bien l'entendre

Chapter Three

The priest stooped[1] on the cobbled churchyard path[2] to pick up a piece of litter[3]: a stray sweet wrapper[4]. He crumpled it in his hand, and stood up slowly to placate the nagging rheumatism[5] in his knee. The pain came from sleeping alone in an old house through many damp Italian winters[6], he knew: but priests ought to be poor. For how could a man be a priest if there was one man in the village who was poorer? The thought was a liturgy of his own invention[7], and by the time he had run through it in his mind[8], the pain had eased[9].

He left the yard to walk across the road to his house[10]. In the middle of the street the rheumatism stabbed him again: a vicious, angry shaft of pain[11] which made him stumble[12]. He made it to the house[13] and leaned on the wall, resting his weight on his good leg.

Looking down the road towards the centre of the village he saw the youngsters whom he had spoken to earlier[14]. They walked very slowly, their arms around each other; looking and smiling at each other. They seemed very much in love – more so than they had half an hour earlier[15]. The understanding which the priest had gained[16] through many years of listening to confessions told him that a change had been wrought[17] in the relationship within the last few minutes. Perhaps it had something to do with their visit to the house of God: maybe he had given them spiritual help, after all.

He had sinned[1], almost certainly, in lying to them[2] about Danielli. The untruth[3] had come automatically, by force of a habit[4] he had got into during the war. Then, when he had felt it imperative[5] to conceal the Jewish family from all enquirers, the whole village had lied with his blessing[6]. To tell the truth would have been sinful.

Today, when a couple of complete strangers had arrived out of the blue[7], and asked for Danielli by name, they had touched an old, raw nerve[8] in the priest; and he had protected the Jews again. The enquiry was bound to be quite innocent: the Fascisti[9] were thirty-five years in the past[10], and no longer worth sinning about. Still, he had not had time to think – which was the reason for most sins, and a poor excuse[11].

He toyed with the idea[12] of going after them, apologizing, explaining, and telling the truth. It would expiate him[13] a little. But there was little point[14]: someone in the village would send them to the bar on the outskirts[15] of Poglio where the Jews eked out their living[16].

His pain had gone. He went into the little house, treading on the loose flagstone[17] at the foot of the stairs with the twinge of affection he reserved for familiar nuisances: like the rheumatism, and the unfailing sins he heard week after week from the irreformable black sheep[18] in his little flock. He gave them a rueful[19] paternal nod of acknowledgement, and granted absolution.

In the kitchen he took out a loaf and cut it with a blunt[20] knife. He found the cheese and scraped off the mould[21]; then he ate his lunch. The cheese tasted good – it was the better for the effect of the mould[22]. There was something he would have not discovered if he had been rich.

1. Il avait péché
2. en leur mentant
3. mensonge
4. poussé par cette habitude
5. lorsqu'il avait senti qu'il était essentiel
6. avait menti avec sa bénédiction
7. à l'improviste
8. touché une vieille corde sensible
9. [mouvement fasciste, fondé par B. Mussolini, 1921]
10. c'était une histoire vieille de trente-cinq ans
11. une mauvaise excuse
12. Il se dit
13. Cela le ferait expier
14. ce n'était pas vraiment nécessaire
15. périphérie
16. gagnaient péniblement leur vie
17. marchant sur la dalle disjointe
18. les irréductibles moutons noirs
19. contrit
20. émoussé
21. racla la moisissure
22. la moisissure l'avait bonifié

1. il essuya l'assiette avec un torchon

2. l'appelaient

3. on savait bien à l'avance

4. rendre visite de façon formelle

5. un homme de petite taille, âgé d'une vingtaine d'années

6. bizarrement vêtu

7. selon les critères du prêtre

8. quelques instants

9. fit entrer l'étranger dans la cuisine rudimentaire

10. poursuivit l'homme, dans un vocabulaire hésitant

11. poursuivaient le même but

12. deux groupes de personnes arrivant

13. c'était trop pour être le seul fruit du hasard

14. Il lui montra les murs nus d'un geste de la main

15. des produits de première nécessité

When he had eaten the meal he wiped the plate with a towel[1] and put it back into the wooden cupboard. The knock at the door surprised him.

People did not usually knock at his door: they opened it and called to him[2]. A knock indicated a formal visit – but in Poglio, one always knew well in advance[3] if someone was going to pay a formal visit[4]. He went to the door with a pleasant sensation of curiosity.

He opened the door to a short man in his twenties[5], with straight fair hair growing over his ears. He was peculiarly dressed[6], by the priest's standards[7], in a businessman's suit and a bow tie. In poor Italian he said: 'Good morning, Father.'

A stranger, thought the priest. That explained the knock. It was most unusual to have so many strangers in the village.

The man said: 'May I talk to you for a few moments[8]?'

'Surely.' The priest ushered the stranger into the bare kitchen[9] and offered him a hard wooden seat.

'Do you speak English?'

The priest shook his head regretfully.

'Ah. Well, I am an art dealer from London,' the man continued haltingly[10]. 'I am looking for old paintings.'

The priest nodded wonderingly. Clearly, this man and the couple in the church were on the same mission[11]. That two sets of people should come[12] to Poglio on the same day looking for paintings was just too much of a coincidence to be credible[13].

He said: 'Well, I have none.' He waved a hand at the bare walls[14] of the room, as if to say that he would buy bare essentials[15] first, if he had any money.

'Perhaps in the church?'

'No, the church has no paintings.'

The man thought for a moment, searching for words[1]. 'Is there a museum in the village? Or perhaps someone with a few paintings in his house?'

The priest laughed. 'My son, this is a poor village. No one buys paintings. In good times[2], when they have a little extra money[3], they eat meat[4] – or perhaps drink wine[5]. There are no art collectors here.'

The stranger looked disappointed. The priest wondered whether to tell him about his rivals[6]. But then he would be forced to mention Danielli, and he would have to give this man information he had withheld from the couple[7].

That seemed unfair[8]. However, he would not lie again. He decided to tell the man about Danielli if he asked: otherwise, he would not volunteer the information[9].

The next question surprised him.

'Is there a family named Modigliani here?'

The priest raised his eyebrows. Quickly, the stranger said: 'Why does the question shock you?'

'Young man, do you really think there is a Modigliani here in Poglio? I am no student of these things[10], but even I know[11] that Modigliani was the greatest Italian painter of this century[12]. It is hardly likely that one of his works lies unnoticed[13] anywhere in the world, let alone Poglio[14].'

'And there is no Modigliani family here,' the man persisted.

'No.'

The man sighed. He stayed in his seat for a moment, staring at the toe of his shoe[15] and wrinkling his brow[16]. Then he stood up.

'Thank you for your help,' he said.

The priest saw him to the door. 'I am sorry I could not give the answers you wanted to hear,' he said. 'God bless you.[17]'

---

1. en cherchant ses mots

2. Lorsque ça va mieux

3. un peu plus d'argent

4. mangent de la viande

5. boivent du vin

6. s'il devait lui parler de ses adversaires

7. une information qu'il avait cachée au couple

8. injuste

9. sinon, il ne lui livrerait pas l'information

10. Bien que je ne connaisse pas le domaine

11. même moi, je sais

12. de notre siècle

13. qu'une de ses œuvres passe inaperçue

14. et encore moins à Poglio

15. le regard rivé sur le bout de ses chaussures

16. fronçant les sourcils

17. Que Dieu vous bénisse.

1. clignant des yeux à la lumière du soleil

2. n'avait probablement jamais appris à prendre soin de lui

3. qu'on leur serve tout sur un plateau d'argent

4. et en plus de ça, il y avait le célibat

5. la fin brutale du sien

6. lorsqu'il avait découvert sa propre virilité

7. mais la simulation n'avait pas duré

8. pour consacrer sa renaissance personnelle

9. ne constituait pas un élément assez solide

10. des pistes incertaines

11. perspective

12. s'était considérablement éloignée

13. Car

14. en l'espace de quelques heures

15. Il était arrivé dans le village par le sud

16. qu'il avait vu

When the door shut behind him, Julian stood outside the priest's house for a moment, blinking in the sunshine[1] and breathing the fresh air. God, the place was smelly. The poor old sod had probably never learned to look after himself[2] – Italian men were used to being waited on hand and foot[3] by their mothers and their wives, he seemed to recall reading.

It was amazing Italy could find enough priests, what with that and the celibacy[4] . . . He grinned as the thought reminded him of the recent abrupt end to his own celibacy[5]. The elation which had come with the discovery of his own potency[6] was still with him. He had proved it had all been Sarah's fault. The bitch had tried to pretend she was not enjoying it at first, but the act had not lasted[7]. What with that, and the sale of her car, and the Modigliani – maybe he was finding his form again.

But he did not have the picture yet. That last stroke of genius was essential, to put the crowning touch to his personal renaissance[8]. The postcard from the girl who signed herself 'D' was a shaky foundation[9] on which to build his hopes, he knew: yet it was by following up dubious leads[10] that great finds were made.

The prospect[11] of the Modigliani had receded a long way[12] during the interview with the priest. If it was here in Poglio it was going to be hard to find. There was one consolation: it looked as if Julian was the first here. For[13] if a painting had been bought in a little place like this, every villager would know about it within hours[14].

He stood beside his rented baby Fiat, wondering what was the next step. He had entered the village from the south[15], and the church was one of the first buildings he had come across[16]. He could look around for a public building: a village hall[1], maybe, or a police station. The priest had said there was no museum.

He decided on a quick reconnaissance[2], and jumped into the little car. Its engine whirred tinnily[3] as he started it and drove slowly into the village. In less than five minutes he had looked at every building. None of them looked promising[4]. The blue Mercedes coupé parked outside the bar must belong to a rich man: the owner obviously did not live in the village.

He drove back to his first parking-spot[5] and got out of the car. There was nothing else for it: he would have to knock on doors. If he went to every house in the village, it could not take all afternoon.

He looked at the small, whitewashed houses: some set back behind kitchen gardens[6], others shoulder-to-shoulder at the roadside[7]. He wondered where to start. Since they were equally improbable[8] places to find a Modigliani, he chose the nearest[9] and walked to the door.

There was no knocker, so he banged on the brown paintwork with his knuckles and waited.

The woman who came to the door had a baby in one arm, its small fist clenched in her unwashed brown hair[10]. Her eyes were set close together[11] about a high, narrow nose[12], giving her a shifty look[13].

Julian said: 'I am an art dealer from England, looking for old paintings. Have you any pictures I could look at, please?'

She stared at him silently for a long minute, a look of disbelief and wariness[14] on her face. Then she shook her head silently and closed the door.

Julian turned away dispirited[15]. He wanted very badly to give up[16] the door-to-door stratagem – it

1. une salle communale
2. Il décida de faire une reconnaissance rapide des lieux
3. vrombit dans un bruit de boîtes de conserve
4. ne semblait prometteur
5. là où il s'était garé au départ
6. en retrait, derrière des potagers
7. côte à côte au bord de la route
8. tout aussi invraisemblables
9. la plus proche
10. dont le petit poing agrippait ses cheveux sales
11. étaient rapprochés
12. au-dessus d'un nez haut et étroit
13. un regard fuyant
14. une expression d'incrédulité et de lassitude
15. découragé
16. Il avait très envie de laisser tomber

made him feel like a salesman[1]. The next house confronted him forbiddingly.[2] Small windows either side of a narrow door reminded him of the face of the woman with the child.

He willed his legs to carry him forward.[3] This door had a knocker: an ornate one, in the shape of a lion's head. The paintwork was new and the windows clean.

A man came, in shirtsleeves[4] and an open waistcoat, smoking a pipe with a badly chewed stem[5]. He was about fifty. Julian repeated his question.

The man frowned; then his face cleared as he penetrated Julian's bad Italian[6]. 'Come in,' he smiled.

Inside, the house was clean and prettily furnished[7]: the floors were scrubbed and the paintwork gleamed[8]. The man sat Julian down.

'You want to see some pictures?' The man spoke slowly and a little too loudly, as if talking to someone who was deaf and senile[9]. Julian assumed his accent was the cause of this. He nodded dumbly[10].

The man raised a finger in a gesture meaning 'Wait' and left the room. He came back a moment later with a pile of framed photographs[11], brown with age and obscured by dust[12].

Julian shook his head. 'I mean paintings,' he said, miming the act of brushing paint on to canvas.

Puzzlement and a trace of exasperation[13] crossed the man's face, and he fingered his moustache[14]. He lifted a small, cheap print of Christ from a nail on the wall and offered it.

Julian took it, pretended to examine it[15], shook his head, and handed it back. 'Any more?'

'No.'

Julian stood up. He tried to put gratitude[16] into his smile. 'I am sorry,' he said. 'You have been kind.'

The man shrugged, and opened the door.

Julian's reluctance to go on was even greater now.[1] Disconsolate and indecisive[2], he stood in the street and felt the hot sun on his neck. He would have to take care not to get burned, he thought inconsequentially.

He considered going for a drink.[3] The bar was a few dozen yards down the road[4], by the blue Mercedes. But a drink would not progress matters[5].

A girl came out of the bar and opened the car door. Julian looked at her. Was she a bitch like Sarah? Any girl rich enough to own one of those had a right to be a bitch. She tossed her hair over one shoulder as she climbed in. The spoiled daughter of a wealthy man[6], Julian thought.

A man came out of the bar and got into the other side of the car, and the girl said something to him. Her voice carried up the street.[7]

Suddenly Julian's mind clicked into gear[8].

He had assumed[9] that the girl was going to drive, but now that he looked more carefully he could see that the steering wheel[10] was on the right-hand side[11] of the car.

The girl's words to the man had sounded like English.

The car had British registration plates[12].

The Mercedes came to life with a throaty chuckle.[13] Julian turned on his heel and walked briskly to where his Fiat was parked. The other car passed him as he keyed the ignition[14], and he did a three-point turn.

A wealthy English girl in a British car in Poglio: it had to be the girl who sent the postcard.

Julian could not take the chance that it was not.

He raced after[15] the Mercedes, letting the tiny engine[16] of the Fiat scream in low gear[17]. The blue car

1. À présent, Julian avait encore moins envie de continuer.

2. Abattu et indécis

3. Il se demanda s'il n'irait pas boire un verre.

4. à quelques dizaines de mètres en contrebas

5. ne ferait pas avancer ses affaires

6. Une fille de riche, pourrie gâtée

7. Sa voix porta jusqu'en haut de la rue

8. se mit en marche

9. Il s'attendait à ce que

10. le volant

11. du côté droit

12. des plaques d'immatriculation anglaises

13. démarra dans un grondement rauque

14. alors qu'il mettait le contact

15. Il se lança à la poursuite

16. petit moteur

17. en première

took a right turn[1], following the west road out of the village. Julian took the same turning[2].

The driver of the Mercedes went fast, handling the powerful car with skill[3]. Julian soon lost the flashing brake-lights[4] in the bends[5] of the lane. He squeezed the last ounce of speed from his car.[6]

When he shot past[7] the Mercedes he almost missed it.[8] He braked to a halt at a crossroads[9] and reversed.

The other car had pulled in off the road[10]. The building it was outside[11] looked at first[12] like a farm-house[13], until Julian saw the beer advertisement in the window.

The young couple had got out and were entering the door to the bar. Julian drove the Fiat in next to their car[14].

On the other side of the Mercedes was a third car; another Fiat, only this was a big, prestige model, painted in a hideous metallic green. Julian wondered who it could belong to.

He got out of his car and followed the others into the bar.

Chapter Four

Peter Usher put down his safety razor[1], dipped his face cloth[2] in hot water and washed the remains of the shaving cream[3] off his face. He studied himself in the mirror.

He picked up a comb[4] and drew his long hair back off his face[5], so that it lay flat above his ears[6] and on top of his head. He combed it carefully down the back of his neck[7] and tucked the long ends[8] under his shirt collar[9].

Without the beard and moustache his face took on a different appearance. His hooked nose[10] and pointed, receding chin[11] gave him the look of a spiv[12], especially with his hair slicked back[13].

He put the comb down and picked up his jacket. It would do. It was only a precaution, anyway.

He walked from the bathroom into the kitchen of the little house. The ten canvases were there, bound in newspapers[14] and tied with string, stacked up against the wall. He stepped around them[15] and went out through the kitchen door.

Mitch's van was parked in the lane at the bottom of the garden. Peter opened the rear doors[16] and wedged them with a pair of planks[17]. Then he began loading the paintings.

The morning was still cool, although the sun was bright and the day promised to be warm. Some of the precautions they were taking were a bit extreme, Peter thought as he lugged[18] a heavy frame down the cracked garden path[19]. Still, it was a good plan:

1. posa son rasoir mécanique

2. trempa son gant de toilette

3. les restes de crème à raser

4. un peigne

5. coiffa ses longs cheveux en arrière

6. pour les aplatir au-dessus des oreilles

7. jusqu'au bas de la nuque

8. rentra les mèches les plus longues

9. col de chemise

10. nez aquilin

11. son menton pointu et fuyant

12. un filou

13. les cheveux lissés en arrière

14. enveloppées dans du papier journal

15. les contourna

16. portières arrière

17. les cala avec deux planches

18. en portant

19. le long de l'allée aux dalles fissurées

dozens of possible snags had been foreseen[1] and taken care of. Each of them was changing his or her appearance slightly[2]. Of course, if it ever came to[3] an identification line-up[4] the disguises would not be enough – but there was no way it could come to that[5].

With the last canvas loaded, he closed the van doors, locked up the house and drove off. He threaded his way[6] patiently through the traffic, resigned to the tedious journey[7] up to the West End.

He found his way to a large college campus[8] in Bloomsbury. He and Mitch had chosen the exact spot a couple of days earlier. The college occupied a block[9] 200 yards wide[10] and almost half a mile long[11]; much of it converted Victorian houses. It had many entrances.

Peter parked on a double yellow line in a little drive which led to one of the college gates. A curious warden would assume he was delivering[12] to the college building beside the gate – but he was on a public road[13], so college officials[14] would not be able to ask him his business[15]. Anyone else would see a young man, presumably a student, unloading junk from an old van.

He opened the rear doors and took the paintings out one by one, leaning them against the railings[16]. When the job was done he closed the van.

There was a telephone box right beside the gates – one of the reasons they had chosen this spot. Peter went in and dialled the number of a taxi firm[17]. He gave his exact location[18], and was promised a cab within five minutes.

It came sooner. The cabbie helped Peter load the canvases into the taxi. They took up most of the back seat.[19] Peter told the driver: 'Hilton Hotel, for a Mr Eric Clapton.' The false name[20] was a joke which had appealed[1] to Mitch. Peter gave the cabbie 50 pence for helping load the paintings, then waved him goodbye[2].

He got into the van when the taxi was out of sight, turned it around, and headed for home. Now there was no way the fakes could be connected with[3] the little house in Clapham.

Anne felt on top of the world[4] as she looked around the suite at the Hilton. Her hair had been styled[5] by Sassoon, and her dress, coat, and shoes came from a madly expensive boutique in Sloane Street. A trace of French perfume was detectable in the air around her.

She lifted her arms and spun around in a circle[6], like a child showing off a party dress[7]. 'If I go to gaol for life[8], this will have been worth it,' she said.

'Make the most of it[9] – those clothes have to be burned tomorrow,' said Mitch. He sat in a plush chair[10] opposite her. His clenched, busy hands betrayed the strain he felt[11] and gave the lie to his easy smile. He was dressed in flared jeans[12], a sweater, and a knitted bobble cap[13], like a faggot playing at being a workman[14], he had said. His hair was piled[15] under the cap to conceal its length, and he wore plastic-rimmed National Health glasses[16] with plain lenses[17].

There was a tentative tap at the door. A room service waiter came in with coffee and cream cakes on a tray.

'Your coffee, madam,' he said, and put the tray down on a low table. 'There is a taxi outside with a number of parcels[18] for you, Mr Clapton,' he added, looking at Mitch.

1. qui avait plu

2. le salua d'un geste de la main

3. les contrefaçons ne pourraient pas être associées à

4. était aux anges

5. Elle s'était fait coiffer

6. exécuta un tour complet sur elle-même

7. qui veut montrer sa belle robe

8. Si je vais en prison à vie

9. Profites-en bien

10. luxueux fauteuil

11. trahissait son stress

12. d'un jean à pattes d'éléphant

13. d'un bonnet de laine à pompon

14. une tapette travestie en ouvrier

15. Ses cheveux étaient rentrés

16. des lunettes à monture en plastique de la sécurité sociale

17. avec des verres neutres

18. des paquets

'Oh, Eric, that will be the paintings. Go and see to it, would you?[1]' Anne spoke in a perfect imitation of French-accented upper-class English[2], and Mitch had to conceal his surprise at the sound.

He went down to the ground floor in the lift, and out through the foyer to the waiting taxi. 'Keep the meter running, chief[3] – madam can afford it[4],' he said.

He turned back to the doorman and pressed two pound notes[5] into his hand. 'See if you can get me[6] a luggage trolley[7], or something, and a helping hand[8],' he said.

The flunkey[9] stepped inside the hotel, and emerged a couple of minutes later with a uniformed bellhop[10] pushing a trolley. Mitch wondered whether any of the tip found its way into the bellhop's pocket[11].

The two of them put five of the paintings on the trolley, and the bellhop disappeared with it. Mitch unloaded the remainder[12] and paid off the cabbie. The empty trolley returned, and Mitch took the rest of the paintings up to the suite. He gave the bell-hop a pound – might as well spread the largesse[13], he thought.

He closed the door and sat down to coffee[14]. He realized that the first stage of the plan had been completed successfully[15]; and with the realization came tension, seeping into his muscles and stringing his nerves tautly[16]. Now there was no turning back[17]. He lit a short cigarette from the packet in his shirt pocket, thinking it would help him relax. It did not – it never did, but he never ceased thinking it would. He tasted his coffee. It was too hot, and he could not summon the patience[18] to wait for it to cool.

He asked Anne: 'What's that?'

She looked up from the clipboard[1] she was scribbling on. 'Our list. Name of the picture, artist, gallery or dealer it's for[2], their phone number, name of the man in charge[3] and his deputy[4].' She scribbled something, then flicked pages in the telephone directory on her lap[5].

'Efficient.' Mitch swallowed his coffee hot, burning his throat. With his cigarette between his lips he began to unpack the paintings.

He piled the discarded newspapers and string[6] in a corner. They had two leather portfolios[7], one large and one small, for taking the works[8] to the galleries. He had not wanted to buy ten, for fear of the purchase being conspicuous[9].

When he had finished, he and Anne sat at the large table[10] in the centre of the room. There were two telephones on it, by request[11]. Anne placed her list by his side[12], and they began phoning.

Anne dialled a number and waited. A girl's voice said: 'Claypole and Company good morning,' all in one breath[13].

'Good morning,' said Anne. 'Mr Claypole, please.' Her French accent had gone[14].

'One moment.[15]' There was a hum, and a click[16], then a second girl.

'Mr Claypole's office.'

'Good morning. Mr Claypole, please,' Anne repeated.

'I'm afraid he's in conference. Who's calling?[17]'

'I have Monsieur Renalle[18] of Agence Arts Nancy. Perhaps Mr de Lincourt is available?'

'If you will hold[19], I'll see.'

There was a pause, and then a male voice[20] came on the line. 'De Lincourt speaking[21].'

'Good morning, Mr de Lincourt. I have Monsieur Renalle of Agence Arts Nancy for you.' Anne nodded

1.	porte–bloc
2.	à qui il est destiné
3.	le responsable
4.	adjoint
5.	sur ses genoux
6.	les restes de papier journal et de ficelle
7.	cartons à dessin en cuir
8.	pour apporter les œuvres
9.	de peur que l'achat ne passe pas inaperçu
10.	prirent place à la grande table
11.	à leur demande
12.	près de lui
13.	d'une seule traite
14.	avait disparu
15.	Un instant.
16.	un bourdonnement suivi d'un clic
17.	C'est de la part de qui ?
18.	M. Renalle est en ligne
19.	Ne quittez pas, s'il vous plaît
20.	une voix masculine
21.	à l'appareil

to Mitch. As she replaced the receiver[1] of her telephone, he lifted his[2].

'Mr de Lincourt?' he said.

'Good morning, Monsieur Renalle.'

'Good morning to you. I am sorry I could not write to you in advance[3], Mr de Lincourt, but my company is representing the estate of a collector[4] and there is a little urgency.' Mitch pronounced 't' with his tongue on the roof of his mouth[5], made 'c' at the back of his throat[6], and softened[7] the 'g' in 'urgency'.

'What can I do to help you?[8]' the dealer asked politely.

'I have a picture which ought to interest you. It's a rather early Van Gogh[9], entitled *The Gravedigger*, seventy-five centimetres by ninety-six. It's rather fine.'

'Splendid.[10] When can we have a look at it?'

'I am in London now, at the Hilton. Perhaps my assistant could pay you a visit this afternoon or tomorrow morning?'

'This afternoon. Shall we say two-thirty?'

'*Bien* – very good. I have your address.'

'Have you a figure in mind[11], Monsieur Renalle?'

'We price the work at about[12] ninety thousand pounds.'

'Well, we can discuss that later.'

'Certainly. My assistant is empowered to come to an agreement[13].'

'I look forward to two-thirty[14], then.'

'Goodbye, Mr de Lincourt.'

Mitch replaced the receiver and sighed heavily.

Anne said: 'God, you're sweating.'

He wiped his forehead[15] with his sleeve. 'I didn't think I'd get to the end of it[16]. That bloody accent[17] – I wish I'd practised more[18].'

'You were marvellous. I wonder what the slimy Mr de Lincourt[1] is thinking right now?'

Mitch lit a cigarette. 'I know. He's delighted to be dealing[2] with a provincial French agent[3] who doesn't know the price of a Van Gogh.'

'The line[4] about representing the estate of a dead collector is great. That makes it plausible that a minor dealer[5] in Nancy should be arranging the sale[6].'

'And he'll be in a hurry to close the deal[7] in case one of his rivals hears about the sucker[8] and gets in first[9].' Mitch smiled grimly. 'Okay, let's do the next[10] on the list.'

Anne picked up the phone and began to dial.

*

The taxi stopped outside the plate-glass windows of Crowforth's in Piccadilly. Anne paid the driver while Mitch lugged the canvas, in its heavy leather case, into the art dealer's splendid premises[11].

A broad, open staircase of Scandinavian pine[12] ran up from the ground-floor showroom[13] to the offices above. Anne led the way up, and knocked on a door.

Ramsey Crowforth turned out to be a wiry, white-haired[14] Glaswegian[15] of about sixty. He peered[16] at Anne and Mitch over his spectacles as he shook hands and offered Anne a seat[17]. Mitch stayed standing, the portfolio clutched in his arms.

His room was panelled[18] in the same pine as the staircase, and his carpet was an orange-brown mixture. He stood in front of his desk, his weight on one foot[19], with one arm dangling[20] at his side and the other on his hip, pushing his jacket back to reveal Lurex[21] braces[22]. He was an authority on[23] the German Expressionists, but he had awful taste, Anne thought.

1. ce mielleux de M. de Lincourt
2. de traiter
3. un agent français établi en province
4. Ta réplique
5. Cela justifie que ce soit un petit marchand
6. qui organise la vente
7. il aura hâte de conclure l'affaire
8. entendrait parler du pigeon
9. le devancerait
10. appelons le prochain
11. les magnifiques locaux du marchand d'art
12. pin de Scandinavie
13. salle d'exposition
14. était un homme aux cheveux blancs frisés
15. originaire de Glasgow
16. Il dévisagea
17. pria Anne de s'asseoir
18. lambrissée.
19. en prenant appui sur un pied
20. un bras ballant d'un côté
21. [fil textile gainé de poly-ester, à l'aspect métallique]
22. bretelles
23. Il faisait autorité dans le domaine

'So you're Mademoiselle Renalle,' he said in his high-pitched Scots[1] accent. 'And the Monsieur Renalle I spoke to this morning was . . .'

'My father,' Anne supplied, avoiding Mitch's eyes.

'Right. Let's see what you've got.[2]'

Anne gestured to Mitch. He took the painting out of the case and stood it on a chair[3]. Crowforth folded his arms[4] and gazed at it.

'An early work,' he said softly[5], speaking as much to himself as the others. 'Before Munch's psychoses really took hold[6]. Fairly typical. . .[7]' He turned away from the picture. 'Would you like a glass of sherry?' Anne nodded. 'And your er . . . assistant?' Mitch declined, with a shake of his head[8].

As he poured, he asked: 'I gather[9] you're acting for the estate of a collector, is that right?'

'Yes.' Anne realized that he was making small talk, to let the impact of the painting sink in[10] before he made a decision. 'His name was Roger Dubois – a businessman. His company made agricultural machinery. His collection was small[11], but very well chosen.'

'Obviously.[12]' Crowforth handed her a glass and leaned back against his desk, studying the picture again. 'This isn't quite my period[13], you know. I specialize in Expressionists in general, rather than Munch in particular: and his early work isn't Expressionist, obviously.' He gestured towards the canvas with his glass.[14] 'I like this, but I would want another opinion on it[15].'

Anne felt a spasm of tension between her shoulders[16], and tried to control the blush which began at her throat[17]. 'I would be happy to leave it with you[18] overnight[19], if you wish,' she said. 'However, there is a provenance.' She opened her briefcase[20] and took out a folder containing the document she had forged[1] back in the studio. It had Meunier's letterhead and stamp.[2] She handed it to Crowforth.

'Oh!' he exclaimed. He studied the certificate. 'This puts a different complexion on matters[3], of course. I can make you an immediate offer.' He studied the picture again for a long moment. 'What was the figure you mentioned this morning?'

Anne controlled her elation. 'Thirty thousand.'

Crowforth smiled, and she wondered whether he, too, was controlling his elation. 'I think we can meet that sum[4].'

To Anne's astonishment, he took a cheque-book[5] from his desk drawer and began to write. Just like that![6] she thought. Aloud she said[7]: 'Would you make it out to[8] Hollows and Cox, our London representatives.' Crowforth looked mildly surprised, so she added: 'They are simply an accounting firm[9], who arrange the transfer of funds[10] to France.' That satisfied him. He tore out the cheque and handed it to her.

'Are you in London long?' he enquired politely[11].

'Just a few days.' Anne was itching to get away[12] now, but she did not want to arouse suspicion[13]. She had to persist with the small talk for the sake of appearances[14].

'Then I hope to see you next time you come.' Crowforth held out his hand.

They left the office and walked down the stairs, Mitch carrying the empty case. Anne whispered excitedly[15]: 'He didn't recognize me!'

'Not surprising. He's only ever seen you from a distance[16]. Besides, then you were the dowdy, mouselike wife[17] of a flamboyant painter. Now you're a vivacious French blonde[18].'

1. qu'elle avait falsifié
2. Il portait l'en-tête et le cachet de Meunier.
3. Voilà qui change la situation
4. que nous pouvons accepter ce montant
5. carnet de chèques
6. C'est aussi simple que ça !
7. À voix haute, elle lui dit
8. Pouvez-vous l'établir à l'ordre de
9. cabinet d'expert-comptable
10. gère le virement des fonds
11. demanda-t-il poliment
12. voulait en finir au plus vite
13. susciter la méfiance
14. pour sauver les apparences
15. chuchota avec excitation
16. de loin
17. l'épouse ordinaire et effacée
18. une Française blonde et dynamique

1. demandèrent au chauffeur de les conduire

2. on a réussi

3. elle se mit à sangloter

4. Déguerpissons d'ici

5. le jour suivant leur installation

6. sac à main en lézard véritable

7. qu'ils avaient laissés un peu partout

8. essuya

9. les surfaces luisantes des meubles

10. Une empreinte isolée

11. ne sera d'aucune utilité

12. le lavabo

13. avant qu'ils pigent

14. il faudrait une vie entière pour toutes les vérifier

15. ils réglaient leur note

16. les toilettes pour dames

17. entra dans une des cabines

18. posa sa valise

19. un imperméable

20. [chapeau de pluie en toile huilée qui descend sur la nuque]

They caught a taxi just outside, and directed the driver[1] to the Hilton. Anne sat back in the seat and looked at the cheque from Crowforth.

'Oh my God, we did it[2],' she said quietly. Then she began to sob[3].

*

'Let's clear out of here[4] as quickly as we can,' said Mitch briskly.

It was one o'clock on the day after they had moved[5] into the Hilton. The last forged masterpiece had just been delivered to a gallery in Chelsea, and there were ten cheques in Anne's genuine lizard-skin handbag[6].

They packed their small suitcases and cleared the room of the pens, papers, and personal possessions they had left around[7]. Mitch took a towel from the bathroom and wiped[8] the telephones and the shiny surfaces of the furniture[9].

'The rest doesn't matter,' he said. 'The odd single print[10] on a wall or a window will be no use at all[11] to the police.' He threw the towel into the sink[12]. 'Besides, there will be so many other prints everywhere by the time they cotton on[13], it will be a life's work sorting them all out[14].'

Five minutes later they checked out[15]. Mitch paid the bill with a cheque on the bank where he had opened the account in the names of Hollows and Cox.

They took a taxi to Harrods. Inside the store they separated. Anne found the ladies'[16] and entered a cubicle[17]. She put her case down[18] on the toilet, opened it, and took out a raincoat[19] and sou'wester-style hat[20]. When she had them on she closed the case and left the cubicle.

200

She looked at herself in the mirror. The coat covered[1] her expensive clothes, and the inelegant hat hid[2] her dyed-blonde hair. A wave of relief swept over her[3] as she realized it no longer mattered whether anyone recognized her[4].

That possibility had kept her on edge[5] right throughout the operation. She did not know any of the people in that stratum[6] of the art world: Peter knew them, of course, but she had always kept out[7] of his relationships with them. She had gone to the odd gallery party[8], where nobody had bothered[9] to speak to her. Still, her face – her normal face – might have been vaguely familiar to someone.

She sighed, and began to clean off[10] her make-up with a tissue[11]. For a day and a half she had been a glamorous woman of the world[12]. Heads had turned as she crossed the street. Middle-aged men had become slightly undignified[13] in her presence, flattering her and opening doors for her. Women had gazed enviously at her clothes.

Now she was back to being[14] – what had Mitch called it? The 'dowdy, mouselike wife of a flamboyant painter'.

She would never be quite the same[15], she felt. In the past she had never been much interested in clothes, make-up and perfume. She had thought of herself as plain[16], and she had been content[17] to be a wife and a mother. Now she had tried the high life[18]. She had been a successful, beautiful villainess[19] – and something hidden, from the depths of her personality[20], had responded to the role. The ghost[21] had escaped from its prison in her heart, and now it would never go back.

She wondered how Peter would react to it.

She dropped the lipstick-stained tissue[22] in a waste-paper basket and left the powder room[23]. She

1. masquait
2. le chapeau ingrat dissimulait
3. Un sentiment de soulagement l'envahit
4. qu'on la reconnaisse
5. l'avait rendue fébrile
6. dans ce milieu
7. elle s'était toujours tenue à l'écart
8. de temps à autre à un cocktail dans une galerie
9. n'avait pris la peine
10. à retirer
11. mouchoir en papier
12. une femme du monde élégante
13. émoustillés, s'étaient montrés un peu moins guindés
14. elle allait redevenir
15. Elle ne serait plus jamais la même
16. quelconque
17. s'était contentée
18. elle avait mené la grande vie
19. criminelle
20. au tréfonds de sa personnalité
21. Le fantôme
22. mouchoir taché de rouge à lèvres
23. toilettes pour dames

left the store by a side entrance. The van was waiting at the kerb, with Peter at the wheel[1]. Mitch was already in the back.

Anne climbed into the passenger seat[2] and kissed Peter.

'Hello, darling,' he said. He started the engine and pulled away from the kerb.

His face was already shadowed with bristles[3]: in a week he would have a respectable beard[4], she knew. His hair fell around his face and down to his shoulders again – the way she liked it.

She closed her eyes and slumped in her seat as they crawled home[5]. The release of tension was a physical pleasure.

Peter pulled up outside a large, detached house[6] in Balham. He went to the door and knocked. A woman with a baby opened it. Peter took the baby and walked back down the path, past the sign which said 'Green-hill Day Nursery[7]', and jumped into the van. He plonked[8] Vibeke on Anne's lap.

She hugged the baby tight.[9] 'Darling, did you miss Mummy[10] last night?'

'Allo,' said Vibeke.

Peter said: 'We had a good time, didn't we, Vibeke? Porridge for tea[11] and cake for breakfast.'

Anne felt the pressure of tears[12], and fought them back[13].

When they arrived home, Peter took a bottle of champagne from the fridge and announced a celebration[14]. They sat around in the studio drinking the sparkling wine[15], giggling as they recalled the worrying moments of the escapade.

Mitch began to fill out a bank deposit slip[16] for the cheques. When he had added up the total he said: 'Five hundred and forty-one thousand pounds, my friends.'

1. au volant
2. grimpa et s'assit sur le siège du passager
3. un duvet recouvrait déjà
4. une barbe tout à fait honorable
5. tandis qu'ils rentraient chez eux au ralenti
6. une grande maison individuelle
7. garderie
8. Il posa
9. Elle serra le bébé très fort
10. Est-ce que maman t'a manqué
11. au goûter
12. sentit les larmes lui monter aux yeux
13. les refoula
14. annonça qu'ils allaient fêter ça
15. le vin pétillant
16. à remplir un bordereau de dépôt

The words seemed to drain Anne's elation.[1] Now she felt tired. She stood up. 'I'm going to dye my hair mouse-coloured again[2],' she said. 'See you later.'

Mitch also stood up. 'I'll go to the bank[3] before they close. The sooner we get these cheques in[4], the better.'

'What about the portfolios?[5]' Peter asked. 'Should we get rid of those?'

'Throw them in the canal tonight,' Mitch replied. He went downstairs, took off his polo-necked sweater, and put on a shirt, tie, and jacket.

Peter came down. 'Are you taking the van?'

'No. Just in case there are small boys taking car numbers[6], I'll go on the tube.' He opened the front door. 'See you.[7]'

It took him just forty minutes to get to the bank in the City. The total on the deposit slip did not even raise the cashier's eyebrows. He checked the figures, stamped the cheque stub[8], and handed the book back to Mitch.

'I'd like a word[9] with the manager, if I may,' Mitch said.

The cashier went away for a couple of minutes. When he came back he unlocked the door and beckoned Mitch[10]. It's that easy to get behind the bulletproof screen[11], Mitch thought. He grinned as he realized he was beginning to think like a criminal. He had once spent three hours arguing with a group of Marxists that crooks were the most militant section of the working class[12].

The bank manager was short, round-faced and genial[13]. He had a slip of paper in front of him with a name and a row of figures[14] on it. 'I'm glad you're making use of our facilities[15], Mr Hollows,' he said to Mitch. 'I see you've deposited over half a million[16].'

---

1. À ces mots, l'exaltation d'Anne sembla retomber.

2. me reteindre les cheveux en gris souris

3. Je vais à la banque

4. Plus nous déposerons ces chèques rapidement

5. Que faisons-nous des cartons à dessin ?

6. des contractuels mettraient des amendes

7. À tout à l'heure.

8. souche

9. Pourrais-je parler

10. lui fit signe d'entrer

11. passer derrière la vitre blindée

12. la fraction la plus militante de la classe ouvrière

13. petit, affable et avait un visage rond

14. une rangée de chiffres

15. que vous ayez recours à nos services

16. plus d'un demi-million

'A business operation that went right[1],' said Mitch. 'Large sums are involved in the art world[2] these days.'

'You and Mr Cox are university teachers, if I remember alright[3].'

'Yes. We decided to use our expertise in the market, and as you can see, it went rather well.'

'Splendid. Well now, is there something else we can do for you?'

'Yes. As these cheques are cleared[4], I would like you to arrange the purchase of negotiable securities[5].'

'Certainly. There is a fee[6] of course.'

'Of course. Spend five hundred thousand pounds on the securities and leave the rest in the account to cover the fee and any small cheques my partner and I have drawn[7].'

The manager scribbled on the sheet of paper.

'One other thing,' Mitch continued. 'I would like to open a safe deposit box[8].'

'Surely. Would you like to see our vault[9]?'

Christ, they make it easy for robbers[10], Mitch thought. 'No, that won't be necessary. But if I could take the key with me now.'

The manager picked up the phone on his desk and spoke into it. Mitch stared out of the window.

'It's on its way[11],' said the manager.

'Good. When you have completed the purchase[12] of securities, put them in the safe deposit.'

A young man came in and handed the manager a key. The manager gave it to Mitch. Mitch stood up and shook hands.

'Thank you for your help.'

'My pleasure[13], Mr Hollows.'

A week later[1] Mitch telephoned the bank and confirmed[2] that the securities had been bought and deposited in the safe. He took an empty suitcase[3] and went to the bank on the tube.

He went down to the vault, opened his box[4], and put all the securities[5] in the suitcase. Then he left.

He walked around the corner to another bank, where he arranged[6] to have another safe deposit box. He paid for the privilege[7] with a cheque of his own[8], and put the new box in his own name[9]. Then he put the suitcase full of securities in the new box.

On the way home he stopped at a phone booth[10] and telephoned a Sunday newspaper[11].

1. Une semaine plus tard
2. pour avoir confirmation
3. une valise vide
4. ouvrit son coffre
5. plaça tous les titres
6. où il fit des démarches
7. régla ce service
8. un de ses chèques personnels
9. mit le nouveau coffre à son propre nom
10. cabine téléphonique
11. journal du dimanche

Chapter Five

Samantha stepped into[1] the Black Gallery and looked around in wonder[2]. The place was transformed.[3] Last time she had been here, it had been full of workmen, rubble, paint cans and plastic sheeting[4]. Now it looked more like an elegant apartment: richly carpeted[5], tastefully decorated, with interesting futuristic furniture[6] and a jungle of bright aluminium spotlights[7] growing out[8] of the low ceiling.

Julian sat at a chrome-and-glass desk[9] just beside the door. When he saw her he got up and shook hands, giving a perfunctory nod to Tom[10].

He said to Sammy: 'I'm thrilled[11] you're going to do the opening for me. Shall I show you around?[12]'

'If you can spare the time from your work[13],' Samantha said politely.

He made a pushing-aside gesture with his hand[14]. 'Just looking at the bills[15], and trying to make them go away by telepathy. Come on.'

Julian had changed, Samantha thought. She studied him as he showed them the paintings and talked about the artists. His earlobe-length fair hair had been layered and styled[16], losing the public-schoolboy look to a more natural, fashionable cut[17]. He spoke now with confidence and authority[18], and his walk was more sure[19] and aggressive. Samantha wondered whether it was the wife problem or the money problem which had been solved: perhaps it was both.

She liked his taste in art[1], she decided. There was nothing breathtakingly original[2] on display – unless you counted the wriggling mass of fibreglas sculpture[3] in the alcove[4] – but the works were modern and somehow well done. The kind of thing I might have on my wall[5], she thought; and found that the expression suited how she felt[6].

He took them around quickly, as if afraid they might get bored. Samantha was grateful: it was all very nice[7], but these days[8] all she wanted to do was get high[9] or sleep. Tom had started to refuse her the pills[10] occasionally, like in the mornings. Without them her moods changed fast[11].

They came full circle[12] to the door. Samantha said: 'I have a favour to ask you, Julian.'

'Your servant, ma'am.[13]'

'Will you get us invited[14] to your father-in-law's house for dinner?'

He raised his eyebrows. 'Why would you want to meet that old shit[15]?'

'He fascinates me. Who would build a million-pound art collection, then sell it? Besides, he sounds like my type[16].' She fluttered her eyelashes.[17]

Julian shrugged. 'If you really want to, it's easy. I'll take you – Sarah and I go to dinner a couple of times a week anyway. It saves cooking.[18] I'll give you a ring.'

'Thank you.'

'Now then, you know that date of the opening. I'd be grateful if you could get here at about six-thirty.'

'Julian, I'm glad to help, but I can't be anything but the last to arrive[19], you know.'

He laughed. 'Of course not. I forget you're a star. The official start is[20] seven-thirty or eight, so perhaps eight o'clock would be best.'

'Okay. But dinner with Lord Cardwell first, right?'

1. ses goûts en matière d'art
2. rien d'original ou à couper le souffle
3. sculpture massive et ondulante en fibre de verre
4. niche
5. que je pourrais accrocher chez moi
6. traduisait bien son état d'esprit
7. c'était beau
8. ces temps-ci
9. se défoncer
10. à lui refuser les comprimés
11. son humeur était instable
12. Ils étaient revenus au point de départ
13. Votre dévoué serviteur, madame.
14. Pouvez-vous nous faire inviter
15. vieux salaud
16. je pense que c'est mon genre d'homme
17. Elle battait des cils.
18. Cela nous évite de faire la cuisine.
19. il faut que j'arrive en dernier
20. Officiellement, cela commence à

'Right.'

They shook hands again. As they left Julian returned to his desk and his bills.

Tom moved sideways through the packed crowd[1] in the street market[2]. It never seemed to be half full: unless it was jammed solid[3] it appeared empty. Street markets were meant to be crowded – the people liked it, and so did the stallholders[4]. Not to mention[5] the pickpockets.

The familiarity of the market[6] made Tom feel uncomfortable. The crockery stall[7], the secondhand clothes[8], the noise, the accents – all represented a world he was glad to have left behind[9]. In the circles he now moved in, he exploited his working-class origins – they were quite fashionable – but he had no fond memories[10]. He looked at the beautiful Asian women[11] in saris, the fat West Indian[12] mothers, the Greek youngsters with their smooth olive skin, the old cockneys in cloth caps, the tired young women with babies, the unemployed lads in the latest stolen bell-bottoms[13]: and he uneasily resisted a sense of belonging[14].

He pushed on through[15] the crowd, aiming for[16] the pub at the end of the street. He heard a singsong voice[17] from a man selling jewellery off an upturned orange crate[18]: 'Stolen property, don't say a word[19]—' He grinned to himself. Some of the goods in the market were stolen, but most of the bargains were just factory rejects[20], too poor in quality to go to the stores. People assumed that if the goods were stolen, they must be good quality.

He came out of the market crowd and entered the Cock. It was a traditional pub: dim, smoky, and slightly smelly[1], with a concrete floor and hard up-right benches[2] along the wall. He went up to the bar.

'Whisky and soda, please. Is Bill Wright here?'

'Old Eyes Wright?' the barman said. He pointed: 'Over there. He's drinking Guinness.'

'One for him, then.'

He paid and carried the drinks to a three-legged table[3] on the far side of the room. 'Morning, Sergeant-Major.'

Wright glared up at him[4] over a pint glass. 'Cheeky young pup[5]. I hope you've bought me a drink.'

'Of course.' Tom sat down. With typical cockney complexity, 'Eyes' Wright's nickname[6] was a double joke: not only was he a former professional soldier[7], but he had bulging eyes of a curious orange colour[8].

Tom sipped his drink and studied the man. The head was shorn to a white bristle[9], except for a small round patch of oiled brown hair[10] right on top. He was deeply tanned, for he spent six weeks every summer and winter in the Caribbean. The money for these holidays he earned as a safe-breaker[11] – the career he had taken up[12] when he had left the Army. He had a reputation for being a skilled workman. He had only been caught once, and that through incredibly bad luck – a burglar had broken[13] into the house Wright was robbing and set off the alarm[14].

Tom said: 'A lovely day for villainry[15], Mr Wright.'

Wright emptied his glass and picked up the one Tom had bought. 'You know what the Bible do say: "The Lord sendeth his sunshine and his rain[16] on the wicked as well as the just[17]." Always been a great consolation to me, that verse.' He drank again. 'You can't be all bad[18], son, if you buy a drink for a poor old man.'

1. sombre, enfumé et sentant un peu mauvais
2. des banquettes raides
3. une table à trois pieds
4. leva les yeux vers lui, d'un air menaçant
5. Petit insolent
6. surnom
7. ancien militaire de profession
8. ses yeux globuleux étaient curieusement orangés
9. tondue pour ne laisser qu'un duvet blanc
10. et un ilot de cheveux bruns huilés
11. perceur de coffres-forts
12. car c'était la carrière qu'il avait choisie
13. un cambrioleur était entré par effraction
14. avait déclenché l'alarme
15. C'est une bonne journée pour les brigands
16. prodigue soleil et pluie
17. aux malfaisants comme aux gentils
18. Tu ne dois pas être si méchant que ça

Tom raised his glass to his lips. 'Good luck.' He reached over and touched Wright's lapel[1]. 'Like the suit.[2] Savile Row?'

'Yes, lad[3]. You know what the Bible do say: "Avoid the *appearance* of evil.[4]" Good advice. Now what copper[5] could bring himself to arrest an old sergeant-major with short hair and a quality suit[6]?'

'Let alone one that could quote the Bible at him[7].'

'Hmmm.' Wright took several large gulps of stout[8]. 'Well, young Thomas, it's about time you stopped beating about the bush.[9] What is it you want?'

Tom lowered his voice. 'I've got a job for you.'

Wright narrowed his eyes. 'What is it?'

'Pictures.'

'Porn?[10] You can't get—'

'No,' Tom interrupted. 'Works of art, you know. Rare stuff.[11]'

Wright shook his head. 'Not my field. I wouldn't know where to get rid[12].'

Tom made an impatient gesture. 'I'm not doing it on my own. I'll need finance anyway.'

'Who's in with you?[13]'

'Well, that's another reason I've come to you. What about Mandingo?[14]'

Wright nodded thoughtfully. 'You're splitting it a lot of ways[15], now. How much is the job worth?'

'A million, all told[16].'

Wright's sandy eyebrows lifted[17]. 'I tell you what – if Mandingo backs it[18], I'm in[19].'

'Great. Let's go see him.'

They left the pub and crossed the road to where a new, mustard-coloured Citroën was parked on a double yellow line. As Wright opened the door, a bearded old man[20] in a stained overcoat[21] came up. Wright gave him some money and got in.

'He looks after the warden[1] for me,' Wright explained as he pulled away. 'You know what the Bible do say: "Do not muzzle the ox[2] that grindeth the corn[3]." Wardens are oxen.'

Tom tried to figure out why the quote was relevant[4] as Wright guided the car south and west. He gave up[5] when they stopped in a narrow street in theatreland[6], near Trafalgar Square.

'He lives here?' Tom said in surprise.

'He does well for himself.[7] "Lo, how the wicked are raised up!" He should be rich, the percentage he takes.[8]' Wright got out of the car.

They went down a narrow street and into a nondescript entrance[9]. A lift took them to the top floor of the building. There was a spyhole[10] in the door Wright knocked on.

It was opened by a dark-skinned young man in matador pants, a loud shirt[11], and beads[12].

Wright said: 'Morning, Mandingo.'

'Hey, man, c'mon in,' said Mandingo. He waved them in[13] with a slim hand from which a long cigarette drooped[14].

The flat was luxuriously decorated in red and black, and cluttered[15] with expensive furniture. The costly electric toys of a man who has more money than he knows how to spend[16] were scattered around: a spherical transistor radio, one large colour TV and another portable one, a digital clock, a mass of hi-fi equipment, and an incongruous antique telephone. A pale blonde girl wearing sunglasses lounged[17] in a deep armchair, a drink in one hand and a cigarette in the other. She nodded at Wright and Tom, and negligently flicked ash[18] on the deep-pile carpet[19].

'Hey, man, what gives[20]?' Mandingo asked as they sat down.

1. les contractuelles
2. Ne muselle pas le bœuf
3. qui moud le blé
4. de comprendre l'allusion
5. renonça
6. quartier des théâtres
7. Il se débrouille très bien.
8. Avec le pourcentage qu'il se prend, c'est normal qu'il soit riche.
9. une entrée tout à fait ordinaire
10. judas
11. une chemise criarde
12. un collier
13. Il les invita à entrer d'un geste
14. d'où pendait une longue cigarette
15. encombré
16. qui a de l'argent à ne savoir qu'en faire
17. se prélassait
18. d'une chiquenaude, envoya sa cendre
19. tapis à poils longs
20. qu'est-ce que vous mijotez

1. voudrait que
tu finances un
petit braquage

2. tu te prends
pour un
dessinateur.

3. Aux
dernières
nouvelles, tu
falsifiais des
chèques.

4. un gros coup

5. amer

6. de minable
falsificateur de
chèques

7. Dis-moi

8. J'ai mes
entrées.

9. si je peux
m'arranger avec
les flics dans ce
quartier

10. tout aura été
cadré à l'avance

11. Une brique

12. Il caressa

13. Alors,
comment ça se
passe ?

14. Il faudra que
je te fournisse

15. deux ou trois
hommes

16. que
j'entrepose ton
précieux butin

17. que je trouve
un marché où
l'écouler

18. pour s'en
débarrasser

19. Note bien

20. pour faire
rentrer l'argent

Wright said: 'Tom here would like you to finance a little blagging[1].'

Tom thought how disparate the two men were, and wondered why they worked together.

Mandingo looked at him. 'Tom Copper, ain't it? So you fancy yourself as a draughtsman.[2] Last I heard you was kiting.[3]'

'This is a big job[4], Mandingo.' Tom was resentful[5]. He did not like to be reminded of his days as a petty cheque-forger[6].

'Give[7], give.'

'You read in the papers about Lord Cardwell's art collection?'

Mandingo nodded.

'I've got an in.[8]'

Mandingo pointed at him. 'I am impressed. Maybe you've come a long way, Tom. Where is it kept?'

'His house in Wimbledon.'

'I don't know if I can fix the police that far out[9].'

'No need,' said Tom. 'There are only thirty paintings. I'll have the whole thing sussed out beforehand[10]. Bill here is working with me. The job will take maybe quarter of an hour.'

Mandingo looked thoughtful. 'A million sobs[11], in fifteen minutes. I like that.' He stroked[12] the blonde girl's thigh absently. 'So what's the deal?[13] You'll want me to supply[14] a van and a couple of labourers[15]; to store the hot stuff[16]; and to find a market for it[17].' He was talking to himself, thinking aloud. 'It'll go to the States. I'll get maybe half a million for it if I do it slowly. Probably take a couple of years to get rid[18].' He looked up. 'Okay. I'll take fifty per cent: you split the other half between you. Bear in mind[19] it'll take a while for the money to come in[20].'

'Fifty per cent?' Tom said. Wright put a restraining hand on his arm.

'Leave it[1], Tom. Mandingo's taking the big risk – storage.'

Mandingo spoke as if he hadn't heard. 'There's something else. You're asking me to put my men at risk[2], lay out money, find storage – even just talking to you I lay myself open[3] to a conspiracy charge[4]. So don't do the job unless you're absolutely certain. If you cock it up[5] – well, just leave the country before I get my hands on you[6]. Failures are bad for my reputation.[7]'

Wright stood up, and Tom followed suit. Mandingo showed them to the door.

He said: 'Hey, Tom, what's your in[8] to that house?'

'I'm going there to dinner. See you.'

Mandingo laughed uproariously[9] as he shut the door.

1. Laisse tomber

2. de faire courir des risques à mes hommes

3. Je m'expose

4. des poursuites pour association de malfaiteurs

5. Si tu merdes

6. avant que je t'attrape

7. Les échecs nuisent à ma réputation.

8. c'est quoi ton entrée

9. éclata de rire

PART FOUR

The Varnish

'I think I know what it is like to be God.'

PABLO PICASSO,
dead painter

Chapter One

The reporter sat at his desk in the newsroom[1], thinking about his career. He had nothing better to do because it was Wednesday, and all decisions made by his superiors on Wednesday were reversed[2] on Thursday morning; therefore[3] he had adopted a policy of never actually working[4] on Wednesdays. Besides, his career offered much food for thought.

It had been a short and spectacular one[5], but there was little substance beneath the glittering surface[6]. He had joined a small weekly[7] in south London after leaving Oxford[8], then he had worked for a news agency[9], then he had managed to get this job[10] on a quality Sunday paper. It had taken him less than five years.

That was the glitter[11]: the dross was that it had been worthless[12]. He had always wanted to be an art critic[13]. That was why he had suffered[14] the weekly in order to learn his trade[15]; and put up[16] with the agency in order to prove his competence[17]. But now, after three months on the Sunday paper, he had realized that he was at the end of a very long queue for the art critic's comfortable chair. There seemed to be no more short cuts[18].

The story he was to do this week involved pollution of a reservoir in South Wales[19]. Today, if anyone asked, he was making preliminary enquiries[20]. Tomorrow the pollution story[21] would have shifted to a beach on the Sussex coast[22], or something[23]. What-

1. dans la salle de rédaction
2. étaient revues
3. c'est pourquoi
4. de ne jamais réellement travailler
5. Jusqu'alors, elle avait été courte et spectaculaire
6. si on grattait le vernis, il n'y avait pas grand-chose
7. un petit hebdomadaire
8. en sortant de l'université d'Oxford
9. une agence de presse
10. son emploi actuel
11. Ça, c'était le vernis
12. le problème, c'était que cela n'avait servi à rien
13. critique d'art
14. il avait enduré
15. afin d'apprendre son métier
16. toléré
17. pour démontrer son talent
18. plus aucun raccourci
19. au sud du Pays de Galles
20. investigations préalables
21. le scénario de pollution
22. une plage de la côte du Sussex
23. ou autre chose

ever happened the job had not the remotest connection[1] with art.

A fat file of newspaper clippings[2] in front of him was marked: 'Water – Pollution – Reservoirs'. He was reaching to open it when the phone rang. He diverted his hand[3] to the receiver.

'Newsdesk.'

'Have you got a pencil ready?[4]'

Louis Broom frowned. He had taken many crank phone calls[5] in five years of journalism, but this approach was a new one[6]. He opened the desk drawer and took out a ballpoint and a pad.

'Yes. What can I do for you?'

The answer was another question. 'Do you know anything[7] about art?'

Louis frowned again. The man did not sound much like[8] a crank. The voice was steady and unhysterical[9], and there was none of the breathless intensity[10] which normally characterized screwball telephoners[11].

'As it happens, I do.[12]'

'Good. Listen carefully, because I won't repeat anything. The biggest fraud in the history of art[13] was perpetrated in London last week.'

Oh dear, thought Louis, it is a crank. 'What is your name, sir?' he said politely.

'Shut up and make a note.[14] Claypole and Company bought a Van Gogh called *The Gravedigger* for eighty-nine thousand pounds. Crowforth's bought a Munch titled *The High Chair* for thirty thousand.'

Louis scribbled frantically[15] as the voice droned a list of[16] ten pictures and galleries.

Finally the voice said: 'The total comes to[17] more than half a million pounds. I'm not asking you to believe me. But you'll have to check. Then, when

218

you've published your story, we will tell you why we did it.'

'Just a minute—' The phone clicked in Louis's ear, and he heard the dial tone[1]. He put the receiver down.

He sat back and lit a cigarette while he wondered what to do about the call. It certainly could not be ignored.[2] Louis was 99 per cent sure the caller was a nutcase[3]: but it was by following up the one-per-centers[4] that great exclusives were found[5].

He debated telling the news editor[6]. If he did, he would probably be told to pass the tip[7] to the art critic. Much better to make a start on the story first, if only to establish his own claim to it[8].

He looked up Claypole in the directory[9] and dialled the number.

'Do you have a Van Gogh called *The Gravedigger* for sale[10]?'

'Just a moment, sir, and I will find out.'

Louis used the pause to light another cigarette.

'Hello? Yes, we do have that work[11].'

'Would you tell me the price?'

'A hundred and six thousand guineas[12].'

'Thank you.'

Louis rang Crowforth & Co. and found that they did indeed have a Munch called *The High Chair* for sale at 39,000 guineas.

He began to think hard[13]. The story was standing up[14]. But it was not yet time[15] to talk about the story.

He picked up the phone and dialled another number.

Professor Peder Schmidt hobbled into the bar on his crutch[16]. He was a big, energetic man with blond hair and a red face. Despite a slight speech

---

1. la tonalité

2. Il ne pouvait en aucun cas passer outre.

3. cinglé

4. en suivant ce fameux un pour cent

5. l'on tombait sur de remarquables exclusivités

6. rédacteur en chef

7. de refiler le tuyau

8. pour pouvoir la revendiquer ensuite

9. dans l'annuaire téléphonique

10. à vendre

11. nous avons bien cette œuvre

12. [ancienne pièce en or, valant 105 pence]

13. à réfléchir très sérieusement

14. se profilait

15. Mais il était prématuré

16. en s'appuyant sur sa béquille

impediment[1] and an atrocious German accent, he had been one of the best art lecturers[2] at Oxford. Although Louis had studied English, he had attended all of Schmidt's lectures for the pleasure of the man's grasp of art history[3] and his enthusiastic, iconoclastic theories. The two men had met outside the lecture theatre[4], gone drinking together, and argued fiercely[5] about the subject closest to their hearts[6].

Schmidt knew more about Van Gogh than any other man alive.

He spotted[7] Louis, waved, and came over.

'The spring[8] on your bloody crutch still squeaks[9],' Louis said.

'Then you can oil it with whisky,' Schmidt replied. 'How are you, Louis? And what is all this secrecy[10] about?'

Louis ordered a large Scotch for the professor. 'I was lucky to catch you[11] in London.'

'You were. Next week I go to Berlin. Everything is hurry and chaos.'

'It was good of you to come.[12]'

'It was indeed. Now what is this about?'

'I want you to look at a picture.'

Schmidt downed[13] his Scotch. 'I hope it's a good one.'

'That's what I want you to tell me. Let's go.'

They left the bar and walked towards Claypole's[14]. The shopping crowds[15] on the West End pavements stared at the odd couple: the young man in his brown chalk-stripe suit and high-heeled shoes[16], and the tall cripple[17] striding along beside him, wearing an open-necked blue shirt and a faded denim jacket. They went along Piccadilly[18] and turned south to St James's. In between an exclusive hatter's[19] and a French restaurant were the leaded bow windows[20] of Claypole's.

They went in and walked the length of the small gallery[1]. At the far end, under a spotlight of its own, they found *The Gravedigger*.

To Louis it was unmistakably[2] a Van Gogh. The heavy limbs[3] and tired face of the peasant, the flat Dutch countryside[4], and the lowering sky[5] were the trademarks[6]. And there was the signature.

'Professor Schmidt! This is an unexpected pleasure[7].'

Louis turned to see a slight, elegant man with a greying Van Dyck beard[8], wearing a black suit. Schmidt said: 'Hello, Claypole.'

Claypole stood beside them[9], looking at the picture. 'Something of a discovery[10], this one, you know,' he said. 'A wonderful picture, but quite new to the market[11].'

'Tell me, Claypole, where did you get it?' Schmidt asked.

'I'm not sure I should tell you. Professional secrets, you know.'

'You tell me where you got it and I will tell you what it is worth[12].'

'Oh, very well. It was a piece of good fortune[13], really. Chap called Renalle, from a minor agency in Nancy[14], was over here last week. Staying at the Hilton and disposing of[15] quite a large collection from the estate of some industrialist or other. Anyway, he simply offered me the picture first[16].'

'And for this you are asking how much?'

'One hundred and six thousand guineas. A fair price[17], I think.'

Schmidt grunted and leaned heavily[18] on his crutch, gazing at the picture.

Claypole said: 'What do you think it's worth?'

Schmidt said: 'About a hundred pounds. It's the best forgery I've ever seen[19].'

1. parcoururent toute la petite galerie
2. sans nul doute
3. Ces membres massifs
4. Ce paysage plat de la campagne hollandaise
5. ce ciel maussade
6. autant de signes distinctifs
7. bonne surprise
8. une barbe grisonnante à la Van Dyck
9. resta près d'eux
10. Une vraie découverte
11. assez nouvelle sur le marché
12. ce qu'elle vaut
13. un coup de chance
14. d'une petite agence de Nancy
15. Il était au Hilton et il voulait liquider
16. Il m'a simplement offert le tableau en premier
17. C'est un bon prix
18. lourdement
19. que j'aie jamais vue

Louis's editor was a short, beak-nosed[1] man with a Northern[2] accent who was fond of the word 'bugger'[3]. He pulled at the end of his nose and said: 'So we know that all of the paintings were bought by the people who the anonymous caller said they were bought by[4]. It seems likely that the prices he mentioned were right. We also know something he didn't tell us: that they were all bought *from* a man calling himself Renalle[5] who was staying at the Hilton. Finally, we know that at least one of the paintings is a forgery.'

Louis nodded. 'The caller also said something like: "We will tell you why we did it." So it sounds as if the caller was in fact Renalle.'

The editor frowned. 'I think it's a stunt[6],' he said.

'That doesn't alter the fact[7] that a mammoth con[8] has been put over on the London art fraternity[9].'

The editor looked up at Louis. 'Don't worry, I'm not knocking the story[10],' he said. He thought for a moment. 'All right, this is how we'll do it.' He turned to Eddie Mackintosh, the paper's art critic. 'I want you to get hold of[11] Disley at the National Gallery, or someone of equal standing[12]. It has to be a body[13] we can call Britain's leading art expert[14]. Get him to go around all these galleries with you and authenticate the pictures or declare them forgeries. Offer a consultancy fee[15] if you think it's wanted.

'Whatever you do, don't tell these guys that their pictures are forgeries. If they find out they'll have the police in. Once the Yard know about it, some hot-shot crime man on a daily[16] will get it and spoil it for us[17].

'Louis, I want you to go at it from the other end[18]. You've got a story[19], whatever Eddie discovers – one major forgery[20] is enough. Try and track down[21] this

Renalle. Find out which room he was in at the hotel, how many people were there, and so on[1]. Okay.'

The tone was dismissive[2], and the two journalists left the editor's office.

Louis gave the reception clerk £5 for a look at the hotel register[3]. There was no Renalle listed for any day the previous week. He double-checked.[4] The only peculiarity[5] was a Mr Eric Clapton. He pointed the name out to the clerk.

'Yes, I remember. He had a beautiful French girl with him. Name something like Renault. I remember, because a taxi came with loads of heavy pictures for him. He was a good tipper[6], too.'

Louis made a note of the room number. 'When guests pay by cheque, do you keep a record of the bank the cheque is drawn on[7]?'

'Yes.'

Louis gave him two more fivers. 'Can you get me the address of this Clapton's bank?'

'Not immediately. Can you come back in half an hour?'

'I'll ring you from my office.'

He walked back[8] to the office to kill the half-hour[9]. When he rang the hotel, the clerk[10] had the answer.

'The cheque was overprinted with the names[11] Hollows and Cox, and Mr Hollows signed it,' he added.

Louis took a taxi to the bank.

The manager told him: 'We never give the addresses of clients, I'm afraid.'

Louis argued: 'These clients have been involved[12] in a major fraud[13]. If you don't give me the addresses now, you'll have to give them to the police soon.'

1. et ainsi de suite

2. Le ton signifia la fin de l'entretien

3. pour jeter un œil sur le registre de l'hôtel

4. Il revérifia.

5. La seule chose étrange

6. Il donnait de généreux pourboires

7. une trace de la banque sur laquelle le chèque est tiré

8. Il rentra à pied

9. pour passer la demi-heure

10. l'employé

11. L'émetteur du chèque était

12. sont impliqués

13. une énorme escroquerie

'When and if the police ask for the addresses, they will get them – provided they have the authority to seize them[1].'

'Would it be compromising yourself to ring them? One of them? And ask their permission?'

'Why should I?'

'I am prepared to remember your help when I write my story. There's no real necessity for the bank to appear in a bad light[2].'

The manager looked thoughtful. After a minute he picked up the phone and dialled. Louis memorized the number.

'There's no reply,' the manager said.

Louis left. From a phone booth he got the operator[3] to put him through[4] to the local exchange for the number[5] the manager had dialled. The local operator gave him the address. He took a taxi.

A station wagon loaded with luggage[6] was parked in the drive. Mr Hollows had just returned from a camping holiday in Scotland with his family. He was untying the ropes on the roof rack[7].

He was worried to find[8] that someone had opened a bank account in his name. No, he had no idea what it could be about. Yes, he could lend[9] Louis a photograph of himself, and he happened to have[10] a snap of himself with his friend Mr Cox.

Louis took the photographs back to the bank[11].

'Neither of those men is the man[12] who opened the account,' said the bank manager.

He was worried now. He telephoned Mr Hollows, and got even more worried[13]. He slipped so far as to tell[14] Louis that a lot of money had passed in and out[15] of the account. It had been converted to negotiable securities, which had been deposited in the bank's safe.

He took Louis to the vault, and opened the safe deposit box Mr Hollows had rented[1]. It was empty.

Louis and the manager looked at each other. Louis said: 'The trail stops here.[2]'

*

'Listen to this: "Britain's top art expert, Mr Jonathan Rand, thinks the paintings are the work[3] of the best art forger[4] this century has seen." Is that you, Mitch, or me?'

Peter and Mitch were sitting in the studio of the Clapham house, drinking the second cup of coffee after breakfast. They had a copy each[5] of the Sunday paper, and they were reading about themselves[6] with a mixture of awe and glee[7].

Mitch said: 'These newspaper boys[8] worked bloody fast[9], you know. They found out all about the bank account and the safe deposit box, and they interviewed poor Hollows.'

'Yes, but what about this: "The forger covered his trail so well[10] that Scotland Yard believe he must have had the help of an experienced criminal[11]." I reckon[12] I'm the brilliant forger and you're the experienced criminal.'

Mitch put the newspaper down and blew on his coffee to cool it[13]. 'It just shows how easily it can be done – which is what we set out to prove.'

'Here's a good bit[14]: "The forger's master-stroke[15] was to provide each painting with a provenance – which is the art world's equivalent of a pedigree[16], and is normally thought to guarantee[17] the authenticity of a work. The provenances were on the official paper of Meunier's, the Paris artists' agents[18], and had the company's stamp[19]. Both paper and stamp must have been stolen." I like that – the master-

1. avait loué
2. La piste s'arrête ici.

3. sont l'œuvre
4. du plus grand faussaire
5. Chacun avait son exemplaire
6. lisaient ce que l'on disait d'eux
7. stupeur et de jubilation
8. Les gars du journal
9. sacrément vite
10. a si bien brouillé les pistes
11. d'un criminel expérimenté
12. J'estime
13. souffla sur son café pour le refroidir
14. un passage intéressant
15. coup de maître
16. l'équivalent d'un pédigree dans le monde de l'art
17. censé garantir
18. l'agent des artistes parisiens
19. portaient le cachet de cette société

stroke.' Peter folded his paper and threw it across the room.

Mitch reached out[1] for Anne's guitar and began to play a simple blues tune[2]. Peter said: 'I hope Arnaz is laughing – he paid for the joke.'

'I don't think he really believed we could pull it off[3].'

'Nor did I,' Peter laughed.

Mitch put the guitar down suddenly, causing the sound-box to boom[4]. 'We haven't done the most important bit yet[5]. Let's get on with it.'

Peter swallowed the rest of his coffee and got up. The two put on their jackets, called goodbye to Anne, and went out.

They walked along the street and squeezed[6] into the telephone booth on the corner.

'Something's worrying me[7],' said Peter as he picked up the phone.

'That bit about Scotland Yard?[8]'

'Right.'

'It's bothering me, too,' said Mitch. 'They might be all set to trace our call[9] to the newspaper. They could get down here to the kiosk, throw a cordon around the area[10], and question everyone[11] until they found someone connected with art.'

'So what do we do?'

'Let's just phone another newspaper. They'll all know about the story by now.'

'Okay.' Peter lifted the directory[12] from the rack and looked under D[13] for Daily[14].

'Which one?' he said.

Mitch closed his eyes and stuck a finger[15] on the page. Peter dialled the number, and asked to speak to a reporter[16].

When he got through[17] he asked: 'Do you take shorthand?[18]'

226

The voice replied testily: 'Of course.'

'Then take.[1] I am Renalle, the master forger[2], and I am about to tell you why I did it. I wanted to prove that the London art scene, in its concentration on master-pieces and dead painters, is phoney. The best ten dealers in London cannot tell a forgery[3] when they see one. They are motivated by greed and snobbery[4], rather than love of art. Because of them the money going into art is diverted away[5] from the artists themselves, who really need it.'

'Slow down,' the reporter protested.

Peter ignored him. 'I am now offering the dealers their money back[6], minus my expenses which come to about one thousand pounds. The condition is that they set aside one-tenth[7] of the cash – that will be about fifty thousand pounds – to provide a building in Central London where young, unknown artists[8] can rent studios at low prices[9]. The dealers must get together[10], and set up a trust fund[11] to buy and manage the building. The other condition is that all police inquiries are dropped[12]. I will look for their reply to my offer in the columns[13] of your newspaper.'

The reporter said quickly: 'Are you a young painter yourself?'

Peter put the phone down.

Mitch said: 'You forgot the French accent.'

'Oh, fuck,' Peter swore[14]. They left the phone booth.

As they walked back to the house, Mitch said: 'What the hell[15], I don't suppose it makes any difference. Now they know it was not a French job[16]. That narrows their field to the whole of the UK. So what?'

Peter bit his lip. 'It shows we're getting slack[17], that's what. We had better be careful not to count our chickens[18] before they've paid up[19].'

1. Alors allez-y
2. maître faussaire
3. ne savent pas reconnaître une contrefaçon
4. Ce sont l'avidité et le snobisme qui les motivent
5. détourné
6. Je propose aux marchands de leur rendre leur argent
7. qu'ils mettent de côté un dixième
8. de jeunes artistes inconnus
9. louer des ateliers à bas prix
10. se réunir
11. constituer un fonds
12. la police doit abandonner toutes les enquêtes
13. les colonnes
14. jura Peter
15. Et puis merde !
16. ce n'était pas l'œuvre de Français
17. nous devenons négligents
18. de ne pas vendre la peau de l'ours
19. avant qu'ils aient payé

1. De l'avoir tué.

2. On les emmerde, les proverbes.

3. Et comment se portent nos joyeux faussaires ?

4. devint livide

5. silhouette trapue

6. avait un paquet sous le bras

7. Tu m'as fait peur

8. le portail en bois vermoulu

9. brandit

10. Je vous félicite, tous les deux

11. J'étais mort de rire

12. fit semblant de regarder les fesses d'Arnaz

13. arrête de délirer

14. Je suis tombé sur le Van Gogh

15. Je suppose que tu ne prends pas de risque

16. si je veux tirer un bénéfice

17. pour rigoler

18. si vous étiez bons

19. Bon sang, où veux-tu en venir

'Hatched.[1]'

'Fuck proverbs.[2]'

Anne was in the front garden, playing with Vibeke in the sunshine, when they got back.

'The sun is shining – let's go out,' she said.

Peter looked at Mitch. 'Why not?'

A deep American voice came from the pavement outside. 'How are the happy forgers?[3]'

Peter whitened[4] and turned around. He relaxed when he saw the stocky figure[5] and white teeth of Arnaz. The man had a parcel under his arm[6].

'You scared me[7],' Peter said.

Still smiling, Arnaz opened the rotting wooden gate[8] and walked in. Peter said: 'Come on inside.'

The three men went up to the studio. When they had sat down Arnaz waved[9] a copy of the newspaper. 'I congratulate you two[10],' he said. 'I couldn't have done a better job myself. I laughed my ass off[11] in bed this morning.'

Mitch got up and pretended to stare at Arnaz's behind[12]. 'How did you get it back on again?'

Peter laughed. 'Mitch, don't get manic again.[13]'

Arnaz went on: 'It was a brilliant operation. And the forgeries were good. I happened to see the Van Gogh[14] in Claypole's last week. I almost bought it.'

'I suppose it's safe for you[15] to come here,' Peter said thoughtfully.

'I think so. Besides, it's necessary if I'm to make a profit[16] on this deal.'

Mitch's voice was hostile. 'I thought you were in this for the laughs[17].'

'That too.' Arnaz smiled again. 'But mainly, I wanted to see just how good the two of you were[18].'

'What the hell are you getting at[19], Arnaz?' Peter was becoming uneasy now.

'Like I said, I want to see a profit on my invest-ment[1]. So I want you to do one more forgery each. For me.'

'No deal[2], Arnaz,' said Peter. 'We did this to make a point[3], not to make money. We're on the verge[4] of getting away with it. No more forgeries.'

Mitch said quietly: 'I don't think we're going to have any choice.'

Arnaz gave him a nod of acknowledgement[5]. He spread his hands in a gesture of appeal[6]. 'Look, you guys, there's no danger. No one will know about these extra forgeries[7]. The people who buy 'em never let on[8] they've been conned[9], because they'll be implicating themselves in something shady[10] by buying them in the first place[11]. And nobody but me will know you did the forging.'

'Not interested,' said Peter.

Arnaz said: 'Mitch knows you're going to do it, don't you, Mitch?'

'Yes, you bastard[12].'

'So tell Pete here.[13]'

'Arnaz has us by the balls[14], Peter,' Mitch said. 'He's the one person in the world who can finger us[15] for the police. All it would take would be one anonym-ous phone call. And we haven't got our deal[16] with the art dealers yet.'

'So? If he fingers us, why can't we finger him?'

Mitch replied: 'Because there's no proof against him[17]. He had no part[18] in the operation – nobody saw him, whereas loads of people[19] saw me. We can be put up on identity parades[20], asked to account for our movements[21] on the day in question, and Christ knows what[22]. All he did was give us money and it was cash, remember? He can deny everything.[23]'

Peter turned to Arnaz. 'When do you want the forgeries?'

1. que mon investissement me rapporte
2. Pas question
3. pour prouver quelque chose
4. sur le point
5. opina de la tête
6. comme s'il les implorait
7. ces nouvelles contrefaçons
8. n'iront jamais raconter
9. qu'ils se sont fait avoir
10. quelque chose de louche
11. les achetant déjà
12. espèce d'enfoiré
13. Alors explique à Pete ici présent.
14. nous tient par les couilles
15. qui peut nous balancer
16. nous n'avons pas conclu notre marché
17. aucune preuve contre lui
18. Il ne faisait pas partie
19. alors que des tonnes de gens
20. séances d'identification
21. qu'on justifie notre emploi du temps
22. Dieu sait quoi encore
23. Il peut tout nier.

'Good lad.[1] I want you to do them now, while I wait.'

Anne looked around the door[2] with the baby in her arms. 'Hey, you lot[3], are we going to the common[4] or not?'

'I'm sorry, darling,' Peter replied. 'It won't be possible now. We've got to do something else.'

Anne's expression was unreadable[5]. She left the room.

Mitch said: 'What sort of paintings do you want, Arnaz?'

The man picked up the parcel he had brought with him. 'I want two copies[6] of this.' He handed it to Mitch.

Mitch unwrapped the parcel[7] and took out a framed painting. He looked at it with puzzlement in his eyes[8]. Then he read the signature[9], and whistled[10].

'Good God[11],' he said in amazement[12]. 'Where did you get this?'

Chapter Two

Samantha toyed with her china coffee cup[1] and watched Lord Cardwell delicately eating[2] a cracker piled high[3] with Blue Stilton[4]. She liked the man, despite herself[5]: he was tall, and white-haired, with a long nose and laugh-lines[6] in the corners of his eyes. Throughout the dinner[7] he had asked her intelligent questions about an actress's work, and had seemed to be genuinely interested[8] – and occasionally scandalized – by the stories she told.

Tom sat opposite her, and Julian at the lower end[9] of the table. The four of them were alone, apart from the butler, and Samantha wondered briefly where Sarah was. Julian had not mentioned her[10]. He was talking enthusiastically now, about a picture he had bought. His eyes shone[11], and he waved his arm in the air as he spoke. Perhaps the picture was the reason for[12] his transformation.

'Modigliani gave it away[13]!' he was saying. 'He gave it to a rabbi in Livorno, who retired to a potty[14] little village in Italy and took it with him. It's been there all these years – hanging on the wall of some peasant's hut[15]!'

'Are you sure it's genuine[16]?' Samantha asked.

'Perfectly. It has characteristic touches[17], it's signed by him, and we know its history. You can't ask more. Besides, I'm having it looked at[18] by one of the top men[19] shortly.'

'It had better be genuine,' Lord Cardwell said. He popped a last crumb of cheese into his mouth[20]

1. tripotait sa tasse à café en porcelaine

2. manger avec délicatesse

3. surmonté de plusieurs tranches

4. [appellation d'origine protégée d'un fromage type « bleu »]

5. Elle ne pouvait s'empêcher d'apprécier cet homme

6. pattes d'oie

7. Pendant tout le dîner

8. de s'intéresser réellement

9. à l'autre extrémité

10. n'en avait pas parlé

11. Ses yeux brillaient

12. était-il à l'origine de

13. l'avait donné

14. perdu

15. de la masure d'un paysan

16. authentique

17. des touches caractéristiques

18. je vais le faire expertiser

19. par une sommité

20. avala un dernier bout de fromage

and sat back in the high dining chair[1]. Samantha watched the butler glide forward[2] and remove his plate. 'It cost us enough money.'

'Us?' Samantha was curious.

'My father-in-law financed the operation,' Julian said quickly.

'Funny – a friend of mine was talking about a lost Modigliani,' Samantha said. She frowned with the effort of remembering[3] – her memory was terrible these days[4]. 'I think she wrote to me about it. Dee Sleign is her name.'

'Must have been another one,' Julian said.

Lord Cardwell sipped his coffee. 'You know, Julian would never have pulled off this great coup of his[5] without some sound advice[6] from me. You won't mind[7] if I tell this story, Julian.'

Samantha guessed he would mind[8], from the look on his face[9], but Cardwell carried on[10].

'He came to me for some money[11] to buy paintings. I told him I'm a businessman, and that if he wants money from me he has to show me how I can make a profit on the deal[12]. I suggested he go away and dig up a real find[13] – then I would risk my money on him. And that's what he did.'

Julian's smile to Samantha implied: 'Let the old fool ramble on.[14]'

Tom said: 'How did you come to be[15] a businessman?'

Cardwell smiled. 'It goes back to my rip-roaring youth[16]. By the time I reached twenty-one[17] I had done just about everything: gone around the world, got sent down from college[18], raced[19] horses and aeroplanes – not to mention[20] the traditional wine, women and song[21].'

He stopped for a moment, gazing into his coffee cup, then went on: 'At the age of twenty-one I came into my money[1], and I also got married. In no time at all, or sooner[2], there was a young 'un on the way[3] – not Sarah, of course, she was much later. All of a sudden I realized that tearing about[4] was a rather limited occupation. And I did not want to manage the estates[5], or work in a firm owned by my father[6]. So I took my money to the City of London, where I discovered no one knew much more about finance than I did. That was about the time the Stock Exchange was falling around everyone's ears[7]. They were all terrified. I bought some companies which, as far as I could see, didn't need to give a toot[8] what happened to the stock market. I was right. When the world got on its feet again, I was four times as rich[9] as I had been at the start. Since then progress has been slower.'

Samantha nodded. It was much as she had guessed. 'Are you glad you went into business[10]?' she asked.

'Not sure.' There seemed to be a note of heaviness in the old man's voice. 'There was a time, you know, when I wanted to change the world, like you young people[11]. I thought I might use my wealth to do somebody some good. But somehow, when you get involved in the business of actually surviving[12], holding companies together[13], satisfying shareholders – you lose interest in such grand schemes[14].'

There was a pause. 'Besides, the world can't be all that bad when there are cigars like these.' He gave a tired smile.[15]

'And pictures like yours,' Samantha put in.

Julian said: 'Are you going to show Sammy and Tom the gallery?'

'Of course.' The old man got up. 'I might as well show 'em off while they're here.[16]'

The butler moved Samantha's chair away[17] as she got up from the table. She followed Cardwell out of

1. j'ai fait un héritage

2. En un rien de temps

3. un bébé en route

4. la dispersion

5. gérer mon patrimoine

6. une société que possédait mon père

7. était en train de s'effondrer

8. à qui il importait peu

9. quatre fois plus riche

10. dans le monde des affaires

11. comme vous, les jeunes

12. survivre au quotidien

13. maintenir vos entreprises à flot

14. vous ne vous intéressez plus à ces grandes idées

15. Il eut un sourire fatigué.

16. autant les exhiber tant qu'ils sont là

17. recula la chaise de Samantha

the dining room into the hall, then up the double staircase[1] to the first floor.

At the top of the stairs Cardwell lifted a large Chinese vase[2] and took a key from under it. Samantha looked sideways at Tom and noticed that he was taking everything in[3], his eyes moving quickly from side to side. Something near the bottom of the doorpost[4] seemed to have caught[5] his attention.

Cardwell opened the stout door[6] and ushered them in. The picture gallery occupied a corner room[7] – probably a drawing room originally[8], Samantha thought. The windows were wire-reinforced[9].

Cardwell showed obvious pleasure as he walked her[10] along the rows of paintings, telling a little about how he had acquired each one.

She asked him: 'Have you always liked paintings?'

He nodded. 'It's one of the things a classical education teaches you[11]. However, there's a lot it leaves out[12] – like the cinema, for example.'

They stopped beside a Modigliani. It was of a naked woman kneeling on the floor – a real woman, Samantha thought, with a plain face[13], untidy hair[14], jutting bones and imperfect skin[15]. She liked it.

Cardwell was such a pleasant, charming man, that she began to feel guilty about planning to rob him. Still, he was losing the pictures anyway, and his insurance would pay up[16]. Besides, the Sheriff of Nottingham was probably quite charming.

She wondered, sometimes, whether she and Tom were slightly mad[17] – whether his madness was an infection he had passed on to her – a sexually transmitted disease[18]. She suppressed a grin. God, she had not felt so alive for years[19].

As they walked out of the gallery she said: 'I'm surprised you're selling the pictures – you seem so fond of them[20].'

Cardwell smiled ruefully. 'Yes. But needs must, when the Devil drives.[1]'

'I know what you mean,' Samantha replied[2].

Chapter Three

'This is bloody awful[1], Willow,' said Charles Lampeth. He felt the language was justified[2]. He had come in to his office on Monday morning, after a weekend in a country house[3] with no telephone and no worries, to find his gallery in the thick of a scandal[4].

Willow stood stiffly[5] in front of Lampeth's desk. He took an envelope from his inside jacket pocket[6] and dropped it on the desk. 'My resignation.[7]'

'There's absolutely no need for it[8],' Lampeth said. 'Every major gallery in London was fooled[9] by these people. Lord, I saw the picture myself and I was taken in[10].'

'It might be better for the gallery if I did go,' Willow persisted[11].

'Nonsense.[12] Now, you've made the gesture and I've refused to accept your resignation, so let's forget it. Sit down, there's a good chap[13], and tell me exactly what happened.'

'It's all in there[14],' Willow replied, pointing at the newspapers[15] on Lampeth's desk. 'The story of the forgery in yesterday's paper, and the terms we're being offered[16] in today's[17].' He sat down and lit a slim cigar.

'Tell me anyway[18].'

'It was while you were in Cornwall[19]. I got a phone call from this chap Renalle, who said he was at the Hilton. Said he had a Pissarro which we might like[20]. I knew we didn't have any Pissarros, of course, so

236

I was quite keen[1]. He came round with the picture that afternoon[2].'

Lampeth interrupted: 'I thought it was a woman who took the pictures to the galleries?'

'Not this one. It was the chap himself.'

'I wonder whether there's a reason for that,' Lampeth mused. 'Anyway, carry on[3].'

'Well, the painting looked good. It looked like Pissarro, it was signed, and there was a provenance from Meunier's. I thought it was worth eighty-five thousand pounds. He asked sixty-nine thousand, so I jumped at it[4]. He said he was from an agency in Nancy, so it seemed quite likely he would under-value a picture[5]. I assumed he was simply not used to handling high-priced works[6]. You came back a couple of days later and approved the purchase, and we put the work on display[7].'

'Thank God[8] we didn't sell it,' Lampeth said fervently. 'You've taken it down, now, of course.'

'First thing this morning.[9]'

'What about this latest development[10]?'

'The ransom[11], you mean? Well, we would get most of our money back. It is humiliating, of course: but nothing compared with the embarrassment of being duped[12] in the first place. And this idea of theirs[13] – low-rent studios for artists – is really quite laudable[14].'

'So what do you suggest?'

'I think the first step must be to get all the dealers together for a meeting[15].'

'Fine.'

'Might we hold it here?'

'I don't see why not. Only get the whole thing over with[16] as soon as possible. The publicity is appalling.[17]'

---

1. alors j'ai manifesté de l'intérêt
2. dans l'après-midi, ce jour-là
3. continuez
4. donc, j'ai sauté sur l'occasion
5. qu'il sous-évalue un tableau
6. de gérer des œuvres de grande valeur
7. nous avons exposé l'œuvre
8. Dieu merci
9. Ce matin à la première heure.
10. ce dernier rebondissement
11. La rançon
12. la honte de s'être fait duper
13. cette idée qu'ils ont eue
14. tout à fait louable
15. organiser une réunion avec tous les marchands d'art
16. finissons-en
17. Toute cette publicité est consternante.

'It will get worse before it improves.[1] The police are coming around later this morning.'

'Then we had better get some work done[2] before they arrive.' Lampeth reached across his desk, lifted the telephone, and said: 'Some coffee, please, Mavis.' He unbuttoned[3] his jacket and put a cigar between his teeth. 'Are we ready for the Modigliani exhibition?'

'Yes. I think it will go well.'

'What have we got?'

'There are Lord Cardwell's three, of course.'

'Yes. They'll be picked up[4] within the next few days.'

'Then we've got the drawings I bought right at the start. They have arrived safely[5].'

'What about dealing pictures[6]?'

'We've done quite well. Dixon is lending us two portraits, the Magi have some sculptures for us, and we've got a couple of oil-and-crayon nudes[7] from Deside's. There are more which I have to confirm.'

'What commission did Dixon want?'

'He asked for twenty-five per cent but I knocked him down to twenty[8].'

Lampeth grunted. 'I wonder why he goes to the trouble[9] of trying it on. Anyone would think[10] we were a shop front[11] in Chelsea instead of a leading gallery[12].'

Willow smiled. 'We always try it on[13] with him.'

'True.'

'You said you had something up your sleeve.'

'Ah, yes.' Lampeth looked at his watch. 'An undiscovered one.[14] I have to go and see about it[15] this morning. Still, it can wait until I've had my coffee[16].'

Lampeth thought about the forger as his taxi threaded its way through the West End towards the City. The man was a lunatic, of course: but a lunatic with altruistic motives[1]. It was easy to be philanthropic[2] with other people's money.

Undoubtedly, the sensible thing would be to give in[3] to his demands. Lampeth just hated to be blackmailed[4].

The cab pulled into the forecourt of the agency and Lampeth entered the building. An assistant helped him with his overcoat[5], which he had worn because of the chill breezes[6] of early September.

Lipsey was waiting for him in his office: the inevitable glass of sherry ready on the table. Lampeth settled his bulk[7] into a chair. He sipped the sherry to warm him.

'So you've got it.'

Lipsey nodded. He turned to the wall and swung aside a section of bookcase[8] to reveal a safe. With a key attached by a thin chain to the waist of his trousers[9], he unlocked the door.

'It's as well[10] I've a big safe,' he said. He reached in with both hands[11] and took out a framed canvas about four feet by three feet[12]. He propped it[13] on his desk where Lampeth could see it, and stood behind it, supporting it[14].

Lampeth stared for a minute. Then he put down his sherry glass, got up, and came closer. He took a magnifier[15] from his pocket and studied the brushwork[16]. Then he stood back and looked again.

'What did you have to give for it?' he asked.

'I'm afraid I forked out[17] fifty thousand pounds.'

'It's worth double that.'

Lipsey moved the painting to the floor and sat down again. 'I think it's hideous[18],' he said.

1. dont le mobile était altruiste

2. de jouer les philanthropes

3. de céder

4. détestait simplement qu'on le fasse chanter

5. lui prit son manteau

6. la brise froide

7. s'installa

8. fit basculer un pan de bibliothèque

9. à la ceinture de son pantalon

10. Cela tombe bien

11. Il plongea ses deux mains à l'intérieur

12. d'environ cent vingt sur quatre-vingt-dix centimètres

13. Il le posa debout

14. se plaça derrière, pour le tenir

15. loupe

16. les coups de pinceau

17. d'avoir dû allonger

18. Je le trouve hideux

'So do I. But it's absolutely unique. Quite astonishing.[1] There's no doubt it's Modigliani – but no one knew he ever painted stuff like this[2].'

'I'm glad you're pleased,' said Lipsey. His tone said he wanted to introduce a more businesslike note[3] into the conversation.

'You must have put a good man[4] on it,' Lampeth mused.

'The best.' Lipsey suppressed a grin. 'He went to Paris, Livorno, Rimini . . .'

'And he beat my niece to it[5].'

'Not exactly. What happened—'

'I don't want to know the details,' Lampeth cut in. 'Have you got a bill ready for me? I'd like to pay it right away.'

'Certainly.' Lipsey went to the office door and spoke to his secretary. He came back with a sheet of paper in his hand.

Lampeth read the bill. Apart from[6] the £50,000 for the painting, it came to £1,904. He took out his personal cheque-book and wrote the amount in[7]. 'You'll get an armoured truck[8] to deliver it?' 'Of course,' Lipsey said. 'That's in the bill[9]. Is everything else satisfactory?'

Lampeth ripped out a cheque and handed it to the detective. 'I consider I've got a bargain[10],' he said.

The New Room was closed to the public, and a long conference table had been brought in and set in the centre[11]. All around the walls were dark, heavy Victorian landscapes[12]. They seemed appropriate to the sombre mood[13] of the men in the room.

The representatives[14] of nine other galleries were there. They sat at the table, while the assistants and solicitors[15] they had brought with them sat in occasional[1] chairs nearby[2]. Willow was at the head of the table[3] with Lampeth beside him. Rain pattered tirelessly[4] against the high, narrow windows in the wall. The air was thick with cigar smoke.[5]

'Gentlemen[6],' Willow began, 'we have all lost a good deal of money and been made to look rather foolish[7]. We cannot retrieve our pride[8], so we are here to discuss getting our money back.'

'It's always dangerous to pay a blackmailer.' The high Scots accent belonged to Ramsey Crowforth. He twanged his braces[9] and looked over the top of his spectacles at Willow. 'If we cooperate with these people, they – or someone else – could try the same stunt again.'

The mild, quiet voice[10] of John Dixon cut in. 'I don't think so, Ramsey. We're all going to be a lot more careful from now on – especially about provenances. This is the kind of trick you can't play twice.[11]'

'I agree[12] with Dixon,' a third man said. Willow looked down the table to see Paul Roberts, the oldest man in the room, talking around the stem of a pipe[13]. He went on: 'I don't think the forger has anything to lose. From what I read in the press, it seems he has covered his tracks so well that the police have little or no hope[14] of finding him, regardless of whether we call them off or not[15]. If we refuse to cooperate, all the villain does is pocket[16] his half a million pounds.'

Willow nodded. Roberts was probably the most respected dealer in London – something of a grand old man[17] of the art world – and his word would carry weight[18].

Willow said, 'Gentlemen, I have made some contingency plans[19] so that, if we do decide to consent to these demands, the thing can be done quickly.'

1. d'appoint
2. à proximité
3. présidait
4. La pluie crépitait inlassablement
5. La fumée des cigares saturait l'atmosphère.
6. Messieurs
7. nous avons été complètement ridiculisés
8. recouvrer notre fierté
9. Il fit claquer ses bretelles
10. La voix douce et posée
11. On ne peut pas jouer deux fois ce genre de tour.
12. Je suis d'accord
13. qui parlait la pipe à la bouche
14. n'ont que peu d'espoir, voire aucun
15. que nous renoncions ou non aux poursuites
16. le malfaiteur n'aura plus qu'à empocher
17. un éminent vieil homme
18. ses arguments auraient du poids
19. j'ai préparé certains plans d'action

He took a sheaf of papers[1] from his briefcase on the floor beside him. 'I've got[2] Mr Jankers here[3], our solicitor, to draw up some papers for the setting up of a trust fund[4].'

He took the top folder from the pile[5] and passed the rest down the table[6]. 'Perhaps you would have a look at these. The important clause[7] is on page three. It says that the trust will do nothing until it receives approximately five hundred thousand pounds from one Monsieur Renalle. At that time[8] it will pay ninety per cent of the money to the ten of us, in proportion to the stated amounts[9] we paid for the forgeries. I think you will find those figures correct.'

Crowforth said: 'Somebody's got to run[10] the trust.'

'I have made some tentative arrangements[11] on that point too,' said Willow. 'They are subject to your approval[12], quite naturally. However, the Principal of the West London College of Art, Mr Richard Pinkman, has agreed to be chairman of the trustees[13] if we so require. I think the vice-chairman should be one of us – perhaps Mr Roberts.

'We would each have to sign a form of agreement[14] withdrawing any claim[15] on the money apart from the arrangement with the trust. And we would have to agree to withdraw our complaint[16] to the police against Monsieur Renalle and his associates[17].'

Crowforth said: 'I want my solicitor to study all these papers before signing anything.'

Willow nodded. 'Of course.'

Roberts said: 'I agree – but all the same[18], we want this business over with[19] quickly. Could we not agree in principle today? The rest could be done by our solicitors over the next day or two, unless there are any snags[20].'

'A good idea,' Willow approved. 'Perhaps our Mr Jankers could coordinate the solicitors' activities?' Jankers bowed his head in acknowledgement.

'Are we all agreed[1], then, gentlemen?' Willow looked around the table for dissenters[2]. There was none. 'All that remains[3], then, is a statement to the press[4]. Will you be happy to leave that with me[5]?' He paused for dissent again. 'Very well. In that case I will release a statement[6] immediately. If you will excuse me, I will leave you in Mr Lampeth's hands. I believe he has organized some tea.'

Willow got up and left the room. He went to his own office and sat down by the telephone. He picked up the receiver – then paused, and smiled to himself.

'I think you've redeemed yourself[7], Willow,' he said quietly.

Willow walked into Lampeth's office with an evening newspaper[8] in his hand. 'It seems it's all over, Lampeth,' he said. 'Jankers has told the press[9] that all the agreements are signed.'

Lampeth looked at his watch. 'Time for a gin[10],' he said. 'Have one?'

'Please.'

Lampeth opened the cabinet and poured gin into two glasses. 'As for its being all over[11], I'm not sure. We haven't got our money yet.' He opened a bottle of tonic[12] and poured half into each glass.

'Oh, we'll get the money. The forgers would hardly have bothered to set this up just to cause trouble. Besides, the sooner they give us the cash, the sooner the police lay off[13].'

'It's not just the money.' Lampeth sat down heavily[14] and swallowed half his drink. 'It will be

1. Tout le monde est-il d'accord
2. en quête de contestataires
3. Nous n'avons plus qu'à faire
4. une déclaration à la presse
5. que je m'en charge
6. Je vais diffuser un communiqué
7. que vous vous êtes racheté
8. journal du soir
9. a informé la presse
10. C'est l'heure de boire un gin
11. Quant au fait que ce soit tout à fait fini
12. [Schweppes®]
13. plus vite la police lâchera l'affaire
14. s'assit péniblement

years before[1] the art world recovers from a blow like this[2]. The public now thinks we're all frauds[3] who don't know the difference between a masterpiece and a seaside postcard[4].'

'I must say, er . . .' Willow hesitated.

'Well?[5]'

'I can't help[6] feeling they have proved a point[7]. Quite what it is I don't know. But something very profound.'

'On the contrary – it's simple. They've proved that the high prices paid for great works of art reflect snobbery[8] rather than artistic appreciation[9]. We all knew that already. They've proved that a real Pissarro is worth no more[10] than an expert copy[11]. Well, it's the public who inflate the price[12], not the dealers.'

Willow smiled and gazed out of the window. 'I know. Still, we make our percentage[13] on the inflation.'

'What do they expect? We couldn't make a living out of fifty-pound canvases.'

'Woolworth's[14] do.'

'And look at the quality of their stuff. No, Willow. The forger may have his heart in the right place, but he won't change anything. We lose prestige for a while – a long while, I expect – but before too long everything will be back to normal, simply because that is the way it has to be.'

'I've no doubt you're right,' said Willow. He finished his drink. 'Well, they're closing up[15] downstairs. Are you ready to go?'

'Yes.' Lampeth stood up, and Willow helped him on with his coat. 'By the way, what did the police say in the paper?'

'They said that since the complaints had been withdrawn[16], they had no option but to suspend enquiries[1]. But they gave the impression they would still like to get hold of Renalle[2].'

Lampeth walked out of the door and Willow followed him. Lampeth said: 'I don't think we'll ever hear from Renalle again.'

The two men were silent as they walked down the stairs and through[3] the empty gallery. Lampeth looked out of the windows and said: 'My car's not here yet. Look at the rain.'

'I'll press on.[4]'

'No, wait. I'll give you a lift.[5] We must talk about the Modigliani exhibition. We haven't had time these last few days.'

Willow pointed across the gallery. 'Somebody's left their shopping,[6]' he said.

Lampeth looked. In a corner, underneath a rather poor charcoal drawing[7], were two large Sainsbury's[8] carrier bags. A carton of soap powder stuck out[9] of the top of one. Willow walked over and looked more closely[10].

He said: 'I suppose we ought to be careful in these days of bag bombs[11]. Do you think the IRA consider us a target?'

Lampeth laughed. 'I don't think they use Fairy Snow in their bombs.' He crossed over the room, and hefted[12] one of the bags.

The wet paper broke[13], and the contents[14] of the bag spilled over the floor[15]. Willow gave a grunt of exclamation and bent down.

Beneath[16] the soap powder and lettuce was a bundle wrapped in newspaper[17]. Inside the newspaper was a pile of stiff cards[18] and sheets of heavyweight paper[19]. Willow sorted through and examined a few.

'They're stocks and bonds[20],' he said finally. 'Open-faced securities[21] – certificates of ownership[22],

1. d'autre choix que d'interrompre l'enquête
2. mettre la main sur Renalle
3. traversaient
4. Bon, je m'en vais.
5. Je vais vous déposer.
6. Quelqu'un a oublié son sac de courses
7. un dessin au fusain plutôt médiocre
8. [chaîne de supermarchés]
9. Une boîte de lessive dépassait
10. regarda de plus près
11. en cette période d'attentats au sac piégé
12. souleva
13. le papier imprégné d'humidité céda
14. le contenu
15. se répandit par terre
16. Sous
17. un paquet enveloppé de papier journal
18. une pile de fiches cartonnées
19. des feuilles de papier épais
20. des actions et des obligations
21. Des titres au porteur
22. certificats de propriété

245

negotiable on signature[1]. I've never seen so much money in all my life.'

Lampeth smiled. 'The forger paid up,' he said. 'The deal is done.[2] I suppose we ought to tell the newspapers.' He stared at the securities for a moment. 'Half a million pounds,' he said quietly. 'Do you realize, Willow – if you snatched those bags[3] and ran away now, you could live well for the rest of your life in South America?'

Willow was about to reply[4] when the gallery door opened.

'I'm afraid we're closed,' Lampeth called out[5].

A man came in. 'It's all right, Mr Lampeth,' he said. 'My name's Louis Broom – we met the other day. I've had a call to say[6] that the half-a-million has been paid back[7]. Is that true?'

Lampeth looked at Willow, and they both smiled. Lampeth said: 'Goodbye, South America.'

Willow shook his head in awe[8]. 'I have to hand it to our friend Renalle.[9] He thought of everything.'

Chapter Four

Julian drove slowly through the quiet Dorset village[1], steering[2] the hired Cortina[3] carefully along the narrow road. All he had by way of an address[4] was Gaston Moore, Dunroamin, Cramford. Dunroamin! It was a mystery how the most discriminating art expert[5] in the country could have called his retirement home[6] such a banal name. Perhaps it was a joke.

Moore was certainly eccentric. He refused to come to London, he had no telephone, and he never answered letters. When the bigwigs[7] of the art world required his services[8], they had to trek down[9] to this village and knock on his door. And they had to pay his fees in crisp one-pound notes[10]. Moore had no bank account.

There never seemed to be anyone around in villages, Julian reflected. He turned a bend[11] and braked hard. A herd of cattle[12] was crossing the road. He killed the engine and got out. He would ask the cowhand[13].

He expected to see a young man with a pudding-basin haircut[14] chewing a stalk of grass[15]. The cowhand was young; but he had a trendy haircut, a pink sweater, and purple trousers tucked into his wellington boots[16].

The man said: 'You lookin' for the painter man?'[17] The accent was a pleasantly rich burr.[18]

'How did you guess?' Julian wondered aloud.

1. ce petit village tranquille du Dorset
2. en conduisant
3. [Ford Cortina]
4. en guise d'adresse
5. l'expert en œuvres d'art le plus averti
6. la maison qu'il avait achetée pour sa retraite
7. les gros bonnets
8. avaient besoin de lui
9. ils devaient se déplacer
10. en billets d'une livre tout neufs
11. Il négocia un virage
12. Un troupeau de vaches
13. vacher
14. une coupe au bol
15. un brin d'herbe
16. un pantalon violet rentré dans ses bottes en caoutchouc
17. Vous cherchez le peintre ?
18. Son accent du terroir était enveloppant et agréable.

'Most furriners want 'un.[1]' The cowhand pointed. 'Back the way you come, turn down the road by the white house. 'Tis a bungalow[2].'

'Thank you.' Julian got back into the car and reversed down the road until he reached the white house. There was a rutted track[3] beside it. He followed the track until he reached a wide gate. 'Dunroamin' was written in faded Gothic lettering[4] on the peeling white paintwork[5].

Julian patted his pocket to make sure the wad of notes[6] was still there; then he took the carefully packed painting from the back seat[7] and manoeuvred it out of the car. He opened the gate and walked up the short path to the door.

Moore's home was a pair of ancient thatched[8] workingmen's cottages[9] which had been knocked into one[10]. The roof was low[11], the windows small and leaded, the mortar between the stones crumbling. Julian would not have called it a bungalow.

His knock was answered, after a long wait, by a bent man with a cane. He had a shock of white hair[12], thick-lensed spectacles[13], and a birdlike tilt to his head[14].

'Mr Moore?' Julian said.

'What if it is?[15]' the man replied in a Yorkshire accent.

'Julian Black, of the Black Gallery. I wonder if you would authenticate[16] a picture for me.'

'Did you bring cash?' Moore was still holding the door, as if ready to slam it[17].

'I did.'

'Come on then.' He led the way inside the house. 'Mind your head[18],' he said unnecessarily – Julian was too short to be bothered by the low beams[19].

The living room seemed to occupy most of one of the cottages. It was crammed with[20] oldish fur-

---

Glossary (left margin):

1. Quand y a des étrangers, c'est souvent pour lui.
2. pavillon
3. un chemin défoncé
4. en lettres gothiques délavées
5. la peinture blanche écaillée
6. liasse de billets
7. siège arrière
8. au toit de chaume
9. [petite maison anglaise traditionnelle, en zone rurale]
10. transformés en une seule habitation
11. Le toit était bas
12. une tignasse blanche
13. des lunettes à double foyer
14. la tête penchée comme celle d'un oiseau
15. Et pour quoi faire ?
16. authentifier
17. comme s'il s'apprêtait à la claquer
18. Attention à la tête
19. poutres basses
20. encombré

niture, among which a brand new[1], very big colour television stuck out like a sore thumb[2]. It smelled of cats and varnish[3].

'Let's have a look at it, then.'

Julian began to unpack the painting, taking off the leather straps[4], the polystyrene sheets[5], and the cotton wool[6].

'No doubt it's another forgery,' Moore said. 'All I see these days is fakes. There's so much of it going on. I see on the telly some smart-alec[7] got them all chasing their behinds[8] the other week. I had to laugh.[9]'

Julian handed him the canvas. 'I think you'll find this one is genuine[10],' he said. 'I just want your seal of approval[11].'

Moore took the painting, but did not look at it. 'Now you must realize[12] something,' he said. 'I can't prove a painting is genuine. The only way to do that is to watch the artist paint it, from start to finish[13], then take it away with you and lock it in a safe. Then you can be sure. All I do is try to prove it's a fake. There are all sorts of ways in which a forgery *might* reveal itself[14], and I know most of them. But if I can find nothing wrong[15], the artist could still turn around[16] tomorrow and say he never painted it[17], and you'd have no argument[18]. Understood?'

'Sure[19],' said Julian.

Moore continued to look at him, the painting face down on his knees[20].

'Well, are you going to examine it?'

'You haven't paid me yet.'

'Sorry.' Julian reached into his pocket for the money.

'Two hundred pounds.'

'Right.' Julian handed over two wads of notes. Moore began to count them.

1. flambant neuve
2. détonnait
3. le chat et le vernis
4. les sangles en cuir
5. les plaques de polystyrène
6. la ouate
7. Je vois à la télé qu'un petit malin
8. tourner en bourrique
9. J'ai bien rigolé.
10. vous constaterez que celui-ci est authentique
11. approbation
12. il faut que vous soyez conscient
13. du début à la fin
14. de débusquer, éventuellement, une contrefaçon
15. je ne trouve rien à redire
16. pourrait malgré tout se manifester
17. déclarer qu'il ne l'a jamais peinte
18. vous n'auriez rien à dire
19. Oui, bien sûr
20. à l'envers sur ses genoux

As he watched, Julian thought how well the old man had chosen to spend his retirement[1]. He lived alone, in peace and quiet[2], conscious of a life's work expertly done[3]. He cocked a snook[4] at the pressures and snobbery of London, giving sparingly of his great skill[5], forcing the art world princes to make a tiresome pilgrimage[6] to his home before he would grant them audience[7]. He was dignified[8] and independent. Julian rather envied him.

Moore finished counting the money and tossed it casually into a drawer[9]. At last he looked at the painting.

Straight away he said: 'Well, if it's a forgery, it's a bloody good one.'

'How can you tell so quickly?'

'The signature is exactly right – not too perfect. That's a mistake most forgers make – they reproduce the signature so exactly it looks contrived[10]. This one flows freely.' He ran his eye over the canvas. 'Unusual. I like it. Well, would you like me to do a chemical test?'

'Why not?'

'Because it means marking the canvas. I have to take a scraping[11]. It can be done in a place where the frame will normally hide the mark[12], but I always ask[13] anyway.'

'Go ahead.'

Moore got up. 'Come along.' He led Julian back through the hallway[14] into the second cottage. The smell of varnish became stronger. 'This is the laboratory,' Moore said.

It was a square room with a wooden workbench[15] along one wall. The windows had been enlarged, and the walls painted white. A fluorescent strip light[16] hung from the ceiling. On the bench were several old paint cans[17] containing peculiar fluids[18].

Moore took out his false teeth[1] with a swift movement[2], and dropped them in a Pyrex beaker[3]. 'Can't work with them in,' he explained. He sat down at his bench and laid the painting in front of him.

He began to dismantle[4] the frame. 'I've got a feeling[5] about you, lad[6],' he said as he worked. 'I think you're like me. They don't accept you as one of them[7], do they?'

Julian frowned in puzzlement. 'I don't think they do.[8]'

'You know, I always knew more about painting than the people I worked for. They used my expertise, but they never really respected me. That's why I'm so bloody-minded with them[9] nowadays. You're like a butler[10], you know. Most good butlers know more[11] about food and wine than their masters. Yet they're still looked down on[12]. It's called class distinction. I spent my life trying to be one of them. I thought being an art expert was the way, but I was wrong. There is no way!'

'How about marrying in?[13]' Julian suggested.

'Is that what you did? You're worse off[14] than me, then. You can't drop out of the race[15]. I feel sorry for you, son.'

One arm[16] of the frame was now free[17], and Moore slid the glass out[18]. He took a sharp knife[19], like a scalpel, from a rack in front of him. He peered closely at the canvas, then delicately ran the blade of the knife across a millimetre of paint.

'Oh,' he grunted.

'What?'

'When did Modigliani die?'

'In 1920.'

'Oh.'

'Why?'

1. dentier
2. d'un geste rapide
3. un gobelet en Pyrex
4. à démonter
5. J'ai un pressentiment
6. mon garçon
7. Ils ne t'admettent pas dans leur cercle
8. Je ne crois pas, non.
9. que je suis si vache avec eux
10. un major-dome
11. s'y connaissent mieux
12. méprisés
13. Et en se mariant dans ce milieu ?
14. Tu es moins bien loti
15. abandonner la course
16. Un des montants
17. était à présent dégagé
18. retira le verre
19. un couteau pointu

'Paint's a bit soft[1], is all. Doesn't mean anything. Hold on.'

He took a bottle of clear liquid from a shelf, poured a little into a test tube[2], and dipped the knife in[3]. Nothing happened for a couple of minutes. To Julian it seemed an age.[4] Then the paint on the knife began to dissolve[5] and seep through[6] the liquid.

Moore looked at Julian. 'That settles it.[7]'

'What have you proved?'

'The paint is no more than three months old[8], young man. You've got a fake. How much did you pay for it?'

Julian looked at the paint dissolving in the test tube. 'It cost me just about everything[9],' he said quietly.

*

He drove back to London in a daze[10]. How it had happened he had no idea. He was trying to figure out[11] what to do about it.

He had gone down to Moore[12] simply with the idea of adding to the value of the painting. It had been a sort of afterthought[13]; there had been no doubt in his mind about the authenticity of the work. Now he wished he had not bothered[14]. And the question he was turning over in his mind, playing with it as a gambler rolls the dice between his palms[15], was: could he pretend[16] he had not seen Moore?

He could still put the picture up in the gallery. No one would know it was not genuine. Moore would never see it, never know it was in circulation.

The trouble was, he might mention it casually[17]. It could be years later. Then the truth would come out[18]: Julian Black had sold a painting he knew to be a fake[19]. That would be the end[20] of his career.

It was unlikely. Good God, Moore would die anyway within a few years[1] – he must be pushing seventy. If only[2] the old man would die soon[3].

Suddenly Julian realized that, for the first time in his life, he was contemplating murder[4]. He shook his head, as if to clear it of confusion. The idea was absurd. But alongside such a drastic notion[5], the risk of showing the picture diminished. What was there to lose? Without the Modigliani, Julian hardly had a career anyway[6]. There would be no more money from his father-in-law, and the gallery would probably be a flop[7].

It was decided, then. He would forget about Moore.[8] He would show[9] the picture.

The essential thing now was to act as if nothing had happened. He was expected for dinner at Lord Cardwell's. Sarah would be there, and she was planning[10] to stay the night. Julian would spend the night with his wife: what could be more normal? He headed for Wimbledon.[11]

When he arrived, a familiar dark blue Daimler[12] was in the drive alongside[13] his father-in-law's Rolls. Julian transferred his fake Modigliani to the boot[14] of the Cortina before going to the door.

'Evening[15], Sims,' he said as the butler opened the door. 'Is that Mr Lampeth's car in the drive?'

'Yes, sir. They are all in the gallery.'

Julian handed over his short coat and mounted the stairs[16]. He could hear Sarah's voice[17] coming from the room at the top.

He stopped short[18] as he entered the gallery. The walls were bare[19].

Cardwell called[20]: 'Come in, Julian, and join in the commiserations[21]. Charles here has taken all my paintings away to sell them.'

---

1. d'ici quelques années

2. Si seulement

3. pouvait mourir bientôt

4. il avait songé au meurtre

5. comparé à cette idée sombre

6. la carrière de Julian ne pèserait pas lourd

7. un échec

8. Moore n'avait jamais existé.

9. exposerait

10. elle avait prévu

11. Il prit la direction de Wimbledon.

12. il reconnut la Daimler bleu foncé

13. qui était garée à côté de

14. le coffre

15. Bonsoir

16. monta l'escalier

17. Il entendit la voix de Sarah

18. Il s'arrêta net

19. étaient nus

20. l'interpella

21. viens t'apitoyer avec nous

Julian walked over, shook hands, and kissed Sarah. 'It's a bit of a shock,' he said. 'The place looks naked.'

'Doesn't it,' Cardwell agreed heartily[1]. 'We're going to have a damn good dinner[2] and forget about it. Sorry, Sarah.'

'You don't have to watch your language[3] with me, you know that,' his daughter said.

'Oh, my God,' Julian breathed[4]. He was staring[5] at one painting left on the wall.

'What is it?' said Lampeth. 'You look as if you've seen a ghost. That's just a little acquisition of mine I brought along[6] to show you all. Can't have a gallery[7] with no pictures at all.'

Julian turned away and walked to the window. His mind was in a turmoil[8]. The picture Lampeth had brought was an exact copy of his fake Modigliani.

The bastard has the real one[9] while Julian had a dud[10]. He almost choked with hatred.[11]

Suddenly a wild, foolhardy plan was born in his mind[12]. He turned around quickly.

They were looking at him, expressions of slightly concerned puzzlement on their faces[13].

Cardwell said: 'I was just telling Charles that you, too, have a new Modigliani, Julian.'

Julian forced a smile. 'That's why this is such a shock. It's exactly like mine.'

'Good Lord!' Lampeth said. 'Have you had it authenticated[14]?'

'No,' Julian lied. 'Have you?[15]'

'Afraid not.[16] Lord, I thought there was no doubt about this one.'

Cardwell said: 'Well, one of you has a forgery. It seems there are more forgeries than genuine works in the art world these days. Personally, I hope

---

Marginal notes:

1. convint vivement Cardwell
2. un bon gueleton
3. Inutile de surveiller ton vocabulaire
4. dit Julian, dans un souffle
5. Il regardait fixement
6. que j'ai apportée
7. Ce n'est pas possible, une galerie
8. en ébullition
9. Ce salaud avait l'original
10. un faux
11. La haine l'empêchait presque de respirer.
12. un plan téméraire et fou lui vint à l'esprit
13. l'air un peu inquiet et perplexe
14. L'avez-vous fait expertiser
15. Et vous ?
16. Non plus.

Julian's is the one[1] – I've got a stake in it.[2]' He laughed heartily.

'They could both be genuine[3],' Sarah said. 'Lots of painters repeated themselves.'

Julian asked Lampeth: 'Where did you get yours?'

'I bought it from a man[4], young Julian.'

Julian realized he had trespassed on the ethics of the profession[5]. 'Sorry,' he mumbled[6].

The butler rang the bell for dinner.

Samantha was flying[7]. Tom had given her the funny little flat tin that evening, and she had taken six of the blue capsules. Her head was light, her nerves tingled[8], and she was bursting with excitement[9].

She sat in the front seat of the van, squashed[10] between Tom and Eyes Wright. Tom was driving. There were two other men in the back.

Tom said: 'Remember, if we're very quiet we should have it off[11] without waxing[12] anybody. If someone does catch us bang to rights[13], pull a shooter on him[14] and tie him up[15]. No violence. Quiet now, we're there.'

He switched the engine off and let the van coast[16] the last few yards. He stopped it just outside the gate of Lord Cardwell's house. He spoke over his shoulder to the men in the back: 'Wait for the word.[17]'

The three in the front got out. They had stocking masks[18], pulled up to their foreheads, ready to cover their faces if they were seen by the occupants of the house.

They walked carefully up the drive. Tom stopped at a manhole[19] and whispered[20] to Wright. 'Burglar alarm.[21]'

1. que celui de Julian est le bon
2. J'y ai une participation.
3. Les deux sont peut-être authentiques
4. Je l'ai acheté à quelqu'un
5. qu'il avait failli à l'éthique du métier
6. marmonna-t-il
7. planait
8. elle avait les nerfs à fleur de peau
9. elle était tout excitée
10. serrée
11. on devrait s'en tirer
12. tuer
13. nous prend sur le fait
14. pointez un flingue sur lui
15. ligotez-le
16. rouler au point mort
17. Attendez le signal.
18. Ils portaient des bas en guise de masque
19. une trappe
20. chuchota
21. Alarme anti-effraction.

Wright bent down and inserted a tool[1] into the man-hole cover. He lifted it easily and shone a pencil torch inside[2]. 'Piece of cake[3],' he said.

Samantha watched, fascinated, as he bent down and put his gloved hands[4] into the tangle of wires[5]. He separated[6] two white ones.

From his little case he took a wire with crocodile clips[7] at either end. The white wires emerged from one side of the manhole and disappeared on the other. Wright clipped the extra wire from his case on to the two terminals[8] on the side of the manhole farthest from the house[9]. Then he disconnected the wires at the opposite pair of terminals. He stood up. 'Direct line to the local nick[10],' he whispered. 'Short-circuited[11] now.'

The three of them approached the house. Wright shone his torch carefully around a window frame[12]. 'Just the one[13],' he whispered. He delved[14] in his bag again and came up with a glass cutter[15].

He cut three sides of a small rectangle in the window near the inside handle[16]. He pulled a strip of tape[17] from a roll and bit it off with his teeth[18]. He wound one end[19] of the tape around his thumb, and pressed[20] the other against the glass. Then he cut the fourth side of the rectangle and lifted the glass out on the end of the tape. He placed it carefully on the ground.

Tom reached through the opening and undid the catch[21]. He swung the window wide and climbed in.

Wright took Samantha's arm and led her to the front door. After a moment it opened silently, and Tom appeared.

The three of them crossed the hall and climbed the stairs. Outside the gallery, Tom took Wright's arm and pointed at the foot of the doorpost.

Wright put down his bag and opened it. He took out an infrared lamp[1], turned it on, and beamed it[2] at the tiny photo-electric cell embedded in the woodwork[3]. With his free hand he took out a tripod[4], set it under the lamp, and adjusted its height[5]. Finally he put the lamp gently[6] on the tripod. He stood up.

Tom took the key from under the vase and opened the gallery door.

Julian lay awake listening to Sarah's breathing. They had decided to stay the night[7] at Lord Cardwell's house after the dinner party. Sarah had been sound asleep[8] for some time. He looked at the luminous hands[9] of his watch: it was 2:30 a.m.

Now was the time.[10] He pulled the sheet off him and sat up slowly, swinging his legs[11] over the edge[12] of the bed. His stomach felt as if someone had tied a knot[13] in it.

It was a simple plan. He would go down to the gallery, take Lampeth's Modigliani, and put it in the trunk of the Cortina. Then he would put the fake Modigliani in the gallery and come back to bed.

Lampeth would never know. The pictures were almost identical. Lampeth would find that his was a fake, and assume that Julian had had the real one all along.

He put on the dressing gown[14] and slippers[15] which had been provided by Sims, and opened the bedroom door.

Creeping around[16] a house at the dead of night[17] was all very well in theory: one thought of how unconscious one would be[18] of anyone else doing it. In reality[19] it seemed full of hazards[20]. Suppose one of the old men got up for the lavatory[21]? Suppose one fell[22] over something?

1. une lampe à infrarouge
2. l'orienta
3. petite cellule photoélectrique encastrée dans le bois
4. trépied
5. en régla la hauteur
6. délicatement
7. de passer la nuit
8. dormait profondément
9. les aiguilles lumineuses
10. C'était le moment ou jamais.
11. en balançant les jambes
12. le bord
13. avait fait un nœud
14. la robe de chambre
15. les pantoufles
16. Circuler à pas de loup
17. au beau milieu de la nuit
18. on se dit qu'on n'entendrait pas
19. Dans les faits
20. un parcours semé d'embûches
21. pour aller aux toilettes
22. Et si on trébuchait

1. Tandis qu'il traversait le palier sur la pointe des pieds
2. si quelqu'un le surprenait
3. se pétrifia
4. quelqu'un murmurer
5. Julian plissa les yeux dans l'obscurité
6. signifiaient qu'il s'agissait de cambrioleurs
7. ils s'étaient fait avoir
8. un faible craquement
9. Il se plaqua
10. une horloge
11. silhouettes
12. traversa un rayon de lune
13. trop stupéfait pour crier
14. pour repérer les lieux
15. comment avait-elle pu s'acoquiner
16. avait mal tourné
17. pour faire face à
18. complète-ment fichu

As he tiptoed along the landing[1] Julian thought of what he would say if he were caught[2]. He was going to compare Lampeth's Modigliani with his own – that would do.

He reached the gallery door and froze[3]. It was open.

He frowned. Cardwell always locked it. Tonight, Julian had watched the man turn the key in the door and put it in its hiding place.

Therefore someone else had got up in the middle of the night to go to the gallery.

He heard a whispered[4]: 'Damn!'

Another voice hissed: 'The bloody things must have been taken away today.'

Julian's eyes narrowed in the darkness[5]. Voices meant thieves[6]. But they had been foiled[7]: the pictures were gone.

There was a faint creak[8], and he pressed himself up[9] against the wall behind a grandfather clock[10]. Three figures[11] came out of the gallery. One carried a picture.

They were taking the real Modigliani.

Julian drew in his breath to shout – then one of the figures passed through a shaft of moonlight[12] from a window. He recognized the famous face of Samantha Winacre. He was too astonished to call out[13].

How could it possibly be Sammy? She – she must have wanted to come to dinner to case the joint[14]! But how had she got mixed up[15] with crooks? Julian shook his head. It hardly mattered. His own plan was awry now.[16]

Julian thought fast to cope with[17] the new situation. There was no longer any need to stop the thieves – he knew where the Modigliani was going. But his own plan was completely spoiled[18].

Suddenly he smiled in the darkness. No, it was not spoiled at all.

A faint breath of cold air[1] told him the thieves had opened the front door. He gave them a minute[2] to get away.

Poor Sammy, he thought.

He went softly down the stairs and out of the open front door[3]. He opened the boot of the Cortina quietly, and took the fake Modigliani out. As he turned back to the house, he saw a rectangle cut in the glass of the dining room window. The window was open. That was how they had got in.

He closed the car boot and went back into the house, leaving the front door open as the thieves had. He climbed to the gallery and hung[4] the fake Modigliani where the real one had been.

Then he went to bed.

He woke early in the morning, although he had slept very little. He bathed[5] and dressed quickly, and went to the kitchen. Sims was already there, eating his own breakfast while the cook[6] prepared the meal for the master of the house and his guests.

'Don't disturb yourself[7],' Julian said to Sims as the butler rose from his seat. 'I'm off early[8] – I'd just like to share your coffee[9], if I may. Cook can see to it.[10]'

Sims piled bacon, egg and sausage on to his fork and finished the meal in one mouthful[11]. 'When one is up early, the rest soon follow, I find[12], Mr Black,' he said. 'I better lay up.[13]'

Julian sat down and sipped his coffee while the butler went away. The shout of surprise came a minute later[14]. Julian had been expecting it[15].

Sims came quickly into the kitchen. 'I think we've been burgled[16], sir,' he said.

1. Un léger courant d'air frais

2. Il laissa passer une minute

3. franchit la porte d'entrée

4. accrocha

5. Il fit sa toilette

6. la cuisinière

7. Ne vous dérangez pas

8. Je pars de bonne heure

9. un peu de café

10. La cuisinière peut s'en charger.

11. en une bouchée

12. c'est ce que j'ai constaté

13. Je ferais bien de dresser la table.

14. survint une minute plus tard

15. s'y attendait

16. que nous avons été cambriolés

Julian faked surprise[1]. 'What?' he exclaimed. He stood up.

'A hole has been cut in the dining room window, and the window is open. I noticed this morning that the front door was open, but I thought Cook had done it. The gallery door was ajar[2], too – but Mr Lampeth's painting is still there.'

'Let's have a look at this window,' said Julian. Sims followed him across the hall and into the dining room.

Julian looked at the hole for a moment. 'I suppose they came for the pictures[3], and were disappointed. They must have decided the Modigliani was worthless[4]. It's an unusual one[5] – they might not recognize it. First thing is to phone the police, Sims. Then rouse Lord Cardwell[6]. Then begin checking[7] the house to see whether anything at all is missing[8].'

'Very good, sir.'

Julian looked at his watch. 'I feel I ought to stay, but I've an important appointment[9]. I think I'll go, as it seems nothing has been taken. Tell Mrs Black[10] I will telephone later.'

Sims nodded and Julian went out.

He drove very fast across London in the early morning. It was windy[11], but the roads were dry. He was guessing that Sammy and her accomplices – who presumably[12] included the boyfriend he had met[13] – would keep[14] the painting at least until today[15].

He stopped outside the Islington house and jumped out of the car, leaving the ignition keys in[16]. There were too many assumptions and guesses[17] in this plan. He was impatient.

He banged hard on the knocker[18] and waited. When there was no reply for a couple of minutes, he banged hard again.

Eventually[1] Samantha came to the door. There was ill-concealed fear in her eyes[2].

'Thank God,' Julian said, and pushed past her[3] into the house.

Tom stood in the hall, a towel around his waist[4]. 'What the hell do you think you're doing, barging—[5]'

'Shut up[6],' Julian said crisply. 'Let's talk downstairs, shall we?'

Tom and Samantha looked at one another[7]. Samantha gave a slight nod[8], and Tom opened the door to the basement stairs[9]. Julian went down.

He sat on the couch and said: 'I want my painting back.[10]'

Samantha said: 'I haven't the faintest idea—[11]'

'Forget it[12], Sammy,' Julian interrupted. 'I know.[13] You broke into[14] Lord Cardwell's house last night to steal his pictures. They were gone, so you stole the one[15] that was there. Unfortunately, it wasn't his[16]. It was mine. If you give it back to me I won't go to the police.'

Silently, Samantha got up and went to a cupboard. She opened the door and took out the painting. She handed it to Julian.

He looked at her face. It was almost haggard: cheeks drawn[17], eyes wide[18] with something which was neither anxiety nor surprise, hair uncared-for[19]. He took the picture from her.

A sense of relief overwhelmed him.[20] He felt quite weak.

Tom would not speak[21] to Samantha. He had been sitting in the chair for three or four hours, smoking, gazing at nothing. She had taken him the cup of coffee Anita made, but it lay cold, untouched[22], on the low table.

1. Au bout d'un moment
2. son regard trahissait la peur
3. entra en la bousculant
4. une serviette autour de la taille
5. Putain, ça va pas de faire irruption...
6. Ferme-la
7. échangèrent un regard
8. lui fit un petit signe de la tête
9. ouvrant sur l'escalier du sous-sol
10. Rendez-moi mon tableau.
11. Mais je n'ai pas la moindre idée...
12. Laisse tomber
13. Je suis au courant.
14. Vous vous êtes introduits
15. le seul
16. il n'était pas à lui
17. ses joues étaient tendues
18. dilatés
19. ses cheveux négligés
20. Un sentiment de soulagement l'envahit.
21. refusait de parler
22. il avait refroidi, intact

She tried again. 'Tom, what does it matter[1]? We shan't be caught[2] – he promised not to go to the police. We've lost nothing. It was just a lark[3], anyway.'

There was no reply.

Samantha laid her head back and closed her eyes. She felt drained[4]; exhausted with a nervous kind of tiredness[5] which would not let her relax. She wanted some pills, but they were all gone. Tom could go out and get her more, if only he would come out of his trance[6].

There was a knock at the front door. At last Tom moved. He looked at the doorway, warily, like a trapped animal[7]. Samantha heard Anita's footsteps along the hall. There was a muted conversation[8].

Suddenly several pairs of feet were coming down the stairs. Tom stood up.

The three men did not look at Samantha.

Two of them were heavily built[9], and carried themselves gracefully like athletes[10]. The third was short. He wore a coat with a velvet collar[11].

It was the short one who spoke. 'You've let the governor down[12], Tom. He's less than pleased. He wants words with you.'

Tom moved fast, but the two big men were faster. As he went for the door, one of them stuck out a foot[13] and the other pushed Tom over it.

They picked him up, each holding an arm. There was a curious, almost sexual smile on the short man's face. He punched Tom's stomach with both fists[14], many times. He carried on long after Tom had slumped[15], eyes closed, in the grip of the other two[16].

Samantha opened her mouth wide[17], but she could not scream.

The little man slapped Tom's face until his eyes opened[18]. The four of them left the room.

Samantha heard the front door slam. Her phone rang. She picked it up automatically[1], and listened.

'Oh, Joe,' she said. 'Joe, thank God you're there[2].' Then she began to cry.

For the second time in two days[3], Julian knocked on the door of Dunroamin. Moore looked surprised when he opened up.

'This time I've got the original,' Julian said.

Moore smiled. 'I hope you have[4],' he said. 'Come in, lad.'

This time he led the way[5] to the laboratory without preamble[6]. 'Give it here[7], then.'

Julian handed the picture over. 'I had a stroke of luck.'

'I'll bet you did.[8] I think you'd better not tell me the details[9].' Moore took out his teeth and dismantled the frame of the painting. 'It looks exactly like yesterday's.[10]'

'Yesterday's was a copy.'

'And now you want the Gaston Moore seal of approval[11].' Moore picked up[12] his knife and scraped[13] a minuscule quantity of paint off the edge of the canvas. He poured the liquid into the test tube and dipped the knife in.

They both waited in silence.

'Looks as though[14] it's all right,' said Julian after a couple of minutes.

'Don't rush.[15]'

They watched again.

'No!' Julian shouted.

The paint was dissolving in the fluid, just like yesterday.

'Another disappointment.[16] I'm sorry, lad.'

1. Elle décrocha machinalement
2. Dieu merci tu es là
3. en deux jours
4. J'espère bien
5. il le conduisit
6. sans préambule
7. Passe-le-moi
8. Je n'en doute pas.
9. qu'il vaut mieux que tu ne m'en dises pas plus
10. Il a l'air identique à celui d'hier.
11. l'approbation de Gaston Moore
12. saisit
13. gratta pour prélever
14. On dirait bien
15. Pas de précipitation.
16. Encore une déception.

Julian banged his fist on the bench[1] in fury. 'How?' he hissed[2]. 'I can't see how!'

Moore put his teeth in again[3]. 'Look here[4], lad. A forgery is a forgery. But no one copies it. Someone's gone to the trouble[5] of making two of these. There's almost certain to be[6] an original somewhere, I reckon[7]. Maybe you could find it. Could you look for it?'

Julian stood up straight. The emotion had washed out of his face[8] now, and he looked defeated[9], yet dignified – as if the battle no longer mattered[10], because he had worked out how it had been lost[11].

'I know exactly where it is,' he said. 'And there's absolutely nothing I can do about it[12].'

Chapter Five

Dee was lying in a sack chair[1], naked, when Mike walked into the Regent's Park flat and shrugged off his coat[2].

'I think it's sexy,' she said.

'It's just a coat,' he replied.

'Mike Arnaz, you are insufferably narcissistic[3],' she laughed. 'I meant the picture.[4]'

He dropped his coat on the carpet and came to sit on the floor beside her. They both gazed at the painting on the wall.

The women were unmistakably[5] Modigliani's women: they had long, narrow faces[6], the characteristic noses, the inscrutable expressions[7]. But that was where the similarity to the rest of his work[8] ended.

They were thrown together in a jumble of limbs and torsos[9], distorted and tangled[10], and mixed up with bits of background[11]: towels, flowers, tables. So far, it prefigured the work Picasso was doing – but keeping secret[12] – in the last years of Modigliani's life. What was different again was the colouring. It was psychedelic: startling pinks[13], oranges, purples, and greens, painted hard and clear[14], quite out of period[15]. The colour bore no relation to the objects coloured[16]: a leg could be green, an apple blue, a woman's hair turquoise.

'It doesn't turn me on[17],' Mike said finally. 'Not that-away[18], anyhow.' He turned away from the pic-

1. un pouf
2. secoua les épaules pour ôter son manteau
3. tu es tellement narcissique
4. Je parlais du tableau.
5. On ne pouvait s'y tromper, ces femmes étaient bien
6. leur visage était long et étroit
7. leur expression énigmatique
8. toute similitude avec le reste de son œuvre
9. dans un fatras de membres et de torses
10. déformées et enchevêtrées
11. fondues dans des fragments d'arrière-plan
12. mais secrètement
13. des roses effrayants
14. appliqués de façon claire et nette
15. sans aucun rapport avec cette période
16. Rien ne reliait les objets à leur couleur
17. Cela ne m'excite pas
18. Pas à cette distance

ture and laid his head on Dee's thigh[1]. 'This, however, does.'

She touched his curly hair with her hand. 'Mike, do you think much about it?'

'Nope.[2]'

'I do. I think what a terrible, loathsome[3], brilliant pair of crooks you and I are. Look what we've got: this beautiful painting, for practically nothing; material for my thesis[4]; and fifty thousand pounds each.' She giggled.

Mike closed his eyes. 'Sure, honey[5].'

Dee shut her eyes, and they both remembered a peasant bar in an Italian village.

Dee entered the bar first, and saw with a shock[6] that the short, dark-haired, dapper[7] man they had sent on a wild goose chase that morning was already there.

Mike thought faster. He hissed in her ear[8]: 'If I leave, keep him talking[9].'

Dee recovered her composure[10] quickly and walked up to the dapper man's table. 'I'm surprised you're still here,' she said pleasantly.

The man stood up. 'So am I,' he said. 'Will you join me?'

The three of them sat around the table. 'What will it be?[11]' the man asked.

'My turn[12], I think,' Mike said. He turned to the back of the bar. 'Two whiskies, one beer,' he called.

'My name is Lipsey, by the way[13].'

'I am Michael Arnaz and this is Dee Sleign.'

'How do you do.' There was a flicker of surprise[14] in Lipsey's eyes at the name[15] Arnaz.

Another man had come into the bar. He looked over at their table.[16]

He hesitated, then said: 'I saw the English number plates. May I join you?'

'I'm Julian Black,' the third man said, and they all introduced themselves.

'It's strange to find so many English people in a little out-of-the-way place like this[1],' Black said.

Lipsey smiled. 'These two are looking for a lost masterpiece,' he said indulgently.

Black said: 'Then you must be Dee Sleign. I'm looking for the same picture.'

Mike cut in quickly.[2] 'And Mr Lipsey is also looking for the picture, although he's the only one who hasn't been candid about it[3].' Lipsey opened his mouth to speak, but Mike forestalled him[4]. 'However, you're both too late[5]. I have the picture already. It's in the trunk of my car. Would you like to see it?'

Without waiting for a reply[6] he got up and left the bar. Dee covered up her astonishment[7] and remembered her instructions.

Lipsey said: 'Well, well, well.'

'Tell me,' Dee said. 'It was only chance[8] that led me to this picture. How did you two get on to it?[9]'

'I'm going to be honest with you,' Black said. 'You wrote a postcard to a mutual friend of ours[10] – Sammy Winacre – and I saw it. I'm setting up[11] my own gallery right now[12], and I couldn't resist the temptation to have a go[13].'

Dee turned to Lipsey. 'So you were sent by my uncle.'

'No,' he said. 'You're quite wrong.[14] I happened to meet[15] an old man in Paris who told me about it[16]. I think he also told you about it.'

There was a shout[17] from the house, and the barman went back to see what it was his wife wanted[18].

1. dans un petit bled aussi paumé

2. l'interrompit abruptement

3. à ne pas l'avoir dit franchement

4. le devança

5. vous arrivez trop tard, l'un et l'autre

6. Sans attendre leur réponse

7. cacha sa stupéfaction

8. C'est simplement le hasard

9. Comment vous êtes-vous lancés là-dedans, vous deux ?

10. une amie commune

11. Je suis en train de monter

12. en ce moment

13. de m'y risquer

14. Vous faites erreur.

15. J'ai rencontré par hasard

16. qui m'en a parlé

17. Ils entendirent un cri

18. ce que lui voulait sa femme

1. ce que pouvait bien mijoter Mike

2. de faire durer la conversation

3. dès lors

4. Je n'avais plus qu'à vous suivre à la trace

5. espérer pouvoir vous doubler

6. Sidérée, Dee vit qu'il avait

7. Puisque vous avez bien failli me devancer

8. doit sortir du pays clandestinement

9. que je dois enfreindre les lois de deux pays

10. à celui d'entre vous

11. dont l'offre est la plus élevée

12. pour annuler une dette de jeu

13. a plus de valeur

14. dans l'annuaire

15. On se reverra à Londres.

Dee wondered what on earth Mike was up to[1]. She tried to keep the conversation going[2]. 'But the old man sent me to Livorno,' she said.

'Me too,' Lipsey acknowledged. 'But by that time[3] all I had to do was follow your trail[4] and hope I might overtake you[5]. I see I failed.'

'Indeed.'

The door opened, and Mike came back in. Dee was flabbergasted to see that he had[6] a canvas under his arm.

He propped it on the table. 'There it is, gentlemen,' he said. 'The painting you came all this way to see.'

They all stared at it.

Eventually Lipsey said: 'What are you planning to do with it, Mr Arnaz?'

'I'm going to sell it to one of you two,' Mike replied. 'Since you so nearly beat me to the punch[7], I will offer you a special deal.'

'Go on,' Black said.

'The point is, this has to be smuggled out of the country[8]. The Italian laws do not permit export of works of art without permission, and if we asked for permission they would try to take it from us. I propose to take the painting to London. This means I have to break the laws of two countries[9] – since I shall have to smuggle it into Britain. In order to cover myself, I will require whichever of you[10] bids highest[11] to sign a piece of paper saying that the money was paid to me to cancel a gambling debt[12].'

'Why won't you sell here?' Black said.

'The painting is worth more[13] in London,' Mike replied with a wide smile. He lifted the painting off the table. 'I'm in the phone book[14],' he said. 'See you in London[15].'

As the blue Mercedes pulled away from the bar and headed for Rimini, Dee said: 'How on earth did you do it?[1]'

'Well, I went around to the back of the bar and spoke to the wife,' Mike said. 'I simply asked her if this was where Danielli stayed[2]*, and she said yes. I asked if he had left any paintings behind, and she showed me this. So I said: "How much do you want for it?*[3]*" That was when she called her husband. He asked for the equivalent of one hundred pounds.'*

'My God!' Dee exclaimed.

'Don't worry,' Mike said. 'I beat him down to eighty.[4]'

Dee opened her eyes. 'After that it was easy,' she said. 'No trouble at Customs[5]. The forgers knocked off a quick couple of copies of the picture for us[6], and both Lipsey and Black paid fifty-thousand-pound gambling debts to us. I haven't got the slightest twinge of conscience[7] about defrauding[8] those two slimy creatures[9]. They would have done the same to us. Especially Lipsey – I'm still sure he was employed by Uncle Charles.'

'Mmmm.' Mike nuzzled Dee.[10] 'Done any thesis today?'

'No. Do you know, I don't think I will do any, ever.'

He raised his head to look at her. 'Why not?'

'After all this, it seems so unreal.'

'What will you do?'

'Well, you once offered me a job.'

'You turned it down.'

'It's different now. I've proved I'm as good as you. And we know we make a team[11], in business as well as in bed.'

---

1. Mais comment as-tu fait ?

2. si c'était là que Danielli avait vécu

3. Combien en voulez-vous ?

4. J'ai marchandé pour qu'il le baisse à quatre-vingts

5. à la douane

6. nous l'ont vite reproduit en deux exemplaires

7. le moindre remords

8. escroqué

9. deux hypocrites

10. Mike caressa Dee du bout du nez.

11. on forme une bonne équipe

'Is this the moment for me to ask you to marry me?'

'No. But there's something else you could do for me.'

Mike smiled. 'I know.' He got up on his knees and kissed her belly, flicking his tongue in and out[1] of her navel[2].

'Hey, there's one thing I haven't figured out[3].'

'Oh, Jesus. Can't you concentrate on sex for a while?'

'Not yet. Listen. You financed those forgers, right? Usher and Mitchell?'

'Yes.'

'When?'

'When I came to London.'

'And the idea was to put them in a position[4] where they had to do the copies for us.'

'Right. Can we screw yet?[5]'

'In a minute.' She pushed his head away[6] from her breasts. 'But when you came to London, you didn't even know I was on the track of the picture.'

'Right.'

'So why did you set the forgers up?[7]'

'I had faith in you[8], baby.'

The room was silent for a while as dusk fell outside[9].

<hr>

1. en faisant des va-et-vient avec la langue

2. nombril

3. que je n'ai pas compris

4. de faire en sorte

5. On peut baiser, maintenant ?

6. Elle repoussa sa tête

7. Alors, pourquoi as-tu piégé les faussaires ?

8. Je te faisais confiance

9. tandis que, dehors, le crépuscule tombait.